BASIC HEALTH PUBLICATIONS

USER'S GUIDE

TO

VITAMINS & MINERALS

Don't Be a Dummy. Become an Expert on What Vitamins & Minerals Can Do for Your Health.

JACK CHALLEM
AND LIZ BROWN

JACK CHALLEM Series Editor

The information contained in this book is based upon the research and personal and professional experiences of the authors. It is not intended as a substitute for consulting with your physician or other health care provider. Any attempt to diagnose and treat an illness should be done under the direction of a health care professional.

The publisher does not advocate the use of any particular health care protocol but believes the information in this book should be available to the public. The publisher and author are not responsible for any adverse effects or consequences resulting from the use of the suggestions, preparations, or procedures discussed in this book. Should the reader have any questions concerning the appropriateness of any procedures or preparation mentioned, the author and the publisher strongly suggest consulting a professional health care advisor.

Series Editor: Jack Challem
Editor: Carol Rosenberg
Typesetter: Gary A. Rosenberg
Series Cover Designer: Mike Stromberg

Basic Health Publications User's Guides are published by Basic Health Publications, Inc.
8200 Boulevard East
North Bergen, NJ 07047
1-800-575-8890

CONTENTS

INTRODUCTION

Vitamins. They captivate. And, yes, they often do cure.

Few newspaper headlines grab a person's attention faster than those describing the seemingly miraculous benefits of vitamins. Almost every week we hear reports that they can reverse heart disease, ease the aches and pains of arthritis, and reduce the risk of cancer.

Vitamins sound almost too good to be true. And you're probably wondering if vitamins are as good as they've been cracked up to be.

The answer, in a nutshell, is a resounding "yes." For years, doctors dismissed the value of vitamins, preferring to prescribe expensive drugs or to perform surgery. Now, each year, medical journals publish thousands of scientific articles describing the health benefits of vitamins, minerals, and other nutrients. And more doctors are recognizing the impressive health benefits of vitamins.

If you're one of the six out of ten Americans who take vitamin supplements, this book will give you a better understanding of how they work to maintain and improve health. If you are thinking about taking vitamins, this book can help you decide what to take.

Vitamins are natural substances found in wholesome foods, and they have many advantages over drugs. They work in tandem with your body to promote health. They're safe. They're relatively inexpensive. They help keep you well. But with all the research and all the confusing headlines on vitamins, it's also easy to be overwhelmed.

This *User's Guide to Vitamins and Minerals* is meant to clear the confusion by providing simple, straightforward answers to your questions about vitamins and minerals. In the first chapter, you'll learn some vitamin basics: why they are important to your health and why supplements are necessary even if you're eating a healthy diet. The following chapters will describe the benefits of specific vitamins or family of vitamins, such as vitamin A; the B vitamins; and vitamins C, D, E, and K.

The second half of this book focuses on minerals, which are nutritionally related to vitamins. Minerals are just as important for health, and you're probably already familiar with at least some of them, such as calcium. You'll also learn about the health benefits of magnesium, chromium, selenium, and other minerals. Finally, the last chapter gives you important tips on how to buy and use vitamins and minerals.

Read on. Be well. And take your vitamins and minerals.

CHAPTER 1

WHAT VITAMINS CAN DO FOR YOUR HEALTH

Your body requires relatively small amounts of vitamins compared with protein or carbohydrate. Still, many people do not obtain enough vitamins, either because they don't eat the right foods or because of absorption problems.

Low levels of vitamins interfere with health, and many people go through life believing their health problems are a normal part of life or aging. When people take vitamin supplements for the first time, they often discover just how dramatically vitamins can improve health.

What Are Vitamins and Minerals?

If you ask a scientist, he or she will tell you that vitamins are organic compounds (containing at least one carbon atom) that promote virtually all biochemical processes in the body. This simple definition actually belies their powerful and diverse roles in health. For example, vitamin C is needed for the formation of skin and all other tissues, as well as for normal functioning of the immune system. Your body cannot make most vitamins, at least not in any substantial amount, so you have to get them from foods or supplements.

In contrast, minerals are elements, meaning that they cannot be broken down into simpler substances. However, minerals that have nutritional roles are found in the form of compounds, meaning they are combined with something else. Calcium citrate and chromium picolinate are examples of the many mineral compounds.

What do vitamins do?
Vitamins initiate and promote virtually all of the body's biochemical activities needed for life and health.

To keep things simple, think of vitamins and minerals as essential ingredients in a recipe—in this case, a recipe for your health. Basically, you need vitamins and minerals to grow, produce energy, fight disease, repair injured tissue, and maintain normal health. Recent scientific studies have even shown that many vitamins and minerals influence the behavior of genes in a positive way. You don't need much of most vitamins and minerals compared with, let's say, dietary protein or carbohydrate. Yet many people do not obtain adequate amounts of these important nutrients.

The thirteen essential vitamins are divided into two groups. One group consists of water-soluble vitamins that need to be replenished daily because they are rapidly excreted. These vitamins include vitamin C and the B-complex family of vitamins.

The second group consists of fat-soluble vitamins, which the body is capable of storing for weeks or months. The fat-soluble vitamins are vitamins A, D, E, and K.

There are also many vitaminlike nutrients that are not officially recognized as vitamins, though their functions are similar. Coenzyme Q_{10}, alpha-lipoic acid, beta-carotene and other carotenoids, and quercetin and other flavonoids are among these vitaminlike nutrients.

You'll learn more about minerals in Chapters 7 through 14.

Vitamins Can Do a Lot for You

Whether you're young or old, male or female, work hard physically or have a desk job, vitamin supplements can often have an amazing effect on your health.

First and foremost, vitamins are essential nutrients that help your body function normally. They can help reduce your risk of developing many serious diseases, such as heart disease, cancer, Alzheimer's disease, and arthritis.

Secondly, many doctors also use vitamins to treat diseases. For example, several large studies with people (not laboratory rats, mind you) have found that vitamin E supplements dramatically reduced the risk of coronary heart disease. Other studies have found that vitamin C reduces symptoms of the common cold and flu by one-third—basically meaning that the vitamin cuts down your sick time by a couple of days.

Still other studies have found that high intake of vitamins reduce the risk of diabetes, arthritis, and many different types of cancer. It practically goes without saying that most people prefer to be healthy than to be sick and miserable. Vitamins can keep you healthy.

One of the most amazing things that happens with vitamin supplementation is what some nutritionally oriented physicians call "side benefits." The term is in sharp contrast to drugs, which tend to have side effects. These doctors have found over and over again that a vitamin supplement prescribed for one condition, such as arthritis, produces unexpected benefits, such as improvements in sleep or mood.

Vitamins Often Reverse Health Problems

Many people who start taking vitamin supplements quickly discover that they can correct and reverse long-standing health problems. For example, British researchers recently gave natural vitamin E supplements (400–800 IU/day) to men and women who had suffered a heart attack. After an average of eighteen months, people getting vitamin E

IU, mg, and mcg
Each is a measurement of vitamins by potency or weight. All three are extremely small amounts. For example, 400 mcg is about $1/70,000$ of an ounce.

had 77 percent fewer heart attacks than those given a dummy pill.

Here's another example: Abram Hoffer, M.D., Ph.D., of Victoria, Canada, has been treating terminal cancer patients with a high-potency vitamin/mineral regimen. He started doing this years ago to treat their depression and anxiety related to the cancer diagnosis. Hoffer has found that 30 percent of his early cancer patients (that is, long-term users of supplements) have lived at least ten years longer than comparable patients who receive only conventional treatment—a phenomenal success rate. So the answer is yes, vitamins can reverse very serious diseases. We'll tell you more about Hoffer's regimen later in this book.

Vitamins Are Good for Healthy People, Too

Vitamins and minerals can certainly correct a lot of damage and reverse or slow the course of many diseases. But you don't have to be a dietitian to figure out that it's far better to prevent diseases. The reason is very simple: it's more difficult to reverse a disease than to prevent it.

You can prevent—or at least reduce the risk of—disease by eating a diet high in fruits and vegetables, exercising, and taking vitamin and mineral supplements. If you're very healthy now, it may take a few years before you see benefits from vitamins. But as the years go by, you'll probably notice that you aren't getting sick as often as people who don't take vitamins and minerals, that your cholesterol and blood pressure aren't creeping up as much as theirs, and that you don't have as many aches and pains.

Are Vitamins a Fountain of Youth?

They may be. Before you dismiss this as too wild of a claim, consider what happens during the aging process. Aging is the result of damage to the 100 trillion cells that compose your body. All of the damage makes these cells less and less efficient with age. An old heart doesn't pump blood as well as a young heart. An old stomach doesn't digest food as well as a young stomach. Old wrinkled skin isn't as supple as baby's skin.

Vitamins function a lot like biological spark plugs that energize your cells and protect them from damage. They promote the myriad biological activities of your cells—and in doing so, they keep them functioning more like younger cells. Numerous studies have shown that vitamin supplements extend life expectancy. Some supplements have age-reversing effects in animals, suggesting that they are likely to have the same effect on people.

Vitamins Are Not the Same as Drugs

Vitamin supplements and drugs might appear similar, but they are very different. Vitamins are not drugs. They are natural substances that should be normally found in the diet, and they work by promoting normal biological processes. Because of poor eating habits (such as too many junk foods or some types of very restrictive diets), many people do not obtain enough vitamins. Scientific studies have found that many people don't consume adequate amounts of vitamins A, C, and E and other nutrients.

In contrast, drugs work by interfering with natural processes in the body, often acting like a chemical sledgehammer to change something. For example, you don't develop a headache because of an aspirin deficiency. However, there are scientific reports showing that vitamin B_2 deficiency can sometimes cause migraine headaches. As another example, antiviral drugs are sometimes used to treat serious viral infections, but these drugs are extremely toxic. In contrast, vitamin C naturally stimulates the activity of the body's own immune cells to fight infections.

Vitamins Are Very Safe

Vitamin supplements are extraordinarily safe. There

are only two vitamins—vitamins A and D—that pose some risk in very high doses because the body stores them. However, it is unlikely that most people will ever overdose on them. The more common problem is that people don't get enough of them.

In general, it's important to follow the usage directions on bottles of these vitamins, which will typically recommend RDA (Recommended Dietary Allowance) or Daily Value (DV) levels of vitamins A and D (5,000 IU and 400 IU, respectively). However, higher doses are often warranted. For example, a recent study, published in the *New England Journal of Medicine*, found that vitamin D deficiency was fairly common among people who seemed to be getting enough of the vitamin. You'll read more about the appropriate uses of high-dose vitamins A and D later in this book.

Vitamins Are More than Catalysts

At one time, doctors and researchers believed that vitamins worked as catalysts to stimulate normal chemical reactions in the body. In chemistry, catalysts promote chemical reactions.

Modern research has changed and broadened this view of vitamins. The building blocks of your body and its biochemicals are nutrients, which include protein, carbohydrate, fats, minerals, and vitamins. In a sense, vitamins help cement together your heart, lungs, skin, brain, and other organs. Vitamins are also needed for your body to make enzymes, hormones, energy, new cells (such as blood and skin cells), and even deoxyribonucleic acid (DNA), which is what your genes are made of.

The latest research on vitamins shows that they protect genes from damage and "turn on" good genes and "turn off" bad genes. The health of your genes is important because they influence your health and your risk of developing cancer. So by helping your body function in a normal way, vitamins enhance health and prevent disease.

You Don't Get Enough Vitamins in Food

We've all heard that Americans are the best fed people in the world. We're also one of the most overfed people in the world, because almost two-thirds of all Americans are now overweight. That situation points to a severe dietary imbalance, and vitamins frequently get shortchanged.

One reason is that many people don't select very nutritious foods. Fruits and vegetables are particularly high in most vitamins, and the U.S. Department of Agriculture recommends that people eat three to five servings of fruits and vegetables daily. Yet several studies have found that only 9 to 32 percent of Americans eat five daily servings of fruits and vegetables, which means that 68 to 91 percent do not! It's easy to be tempted by burgers, fries, fried chicken, and super-sized drinks—and to skip salads and broccoli—and to miss a lot of vitamins.

Another reason people often don't get enough vitamins is that the American diet has undergone tremendous changes in processing over the past 100 years. In the nineteenth century, people ate whole-grain breads rich in vitamin E. Around 1900, technological changes in the milling of grains removed the vitamins, leaving white starch for bread making. Even though bread is "enriched" with a few vitamins, far more nutrients are removed from bread than are added back in.

In addition, soils deficient in some minerals limit a plant's production of vitamins. Synthetic fertilizers (in contrast to plain old manure) don't solve the problem. Several years ago, U.S. Department of Agriculture researchers found that conventional nitrogen fertilizer reduced vitamin C levels in some food crops by as much as one third. Additional nutrient losses have been documented during the transportation, storage, and processing of produce and during cooking. So even if your intentions are good, it's often hard to buy nutritious foods.

The Average Diet Is Pretty Bad

Nutritional surveys have found that half of Americans consume less than 50 mg and 25 percent consume less than 39 mg of vitamin C daily—far below the Recommended Dietary Allowance (RDA) of 90 mg. Other studies have found that half of the population consumes only 950 IU of vitamin A (19 percent of the RDA) and 4 IU of vitamin E (18 percent of the RDA) or less daily.

The same pattern applies to the consumption of other micronutrients as well, meaning that large numbers of people simply aren't getting enough vitamins. These numbers look even worse if you consider that the RDA is a very conservative number, and that typical requirements are probably higher.

Furthermore, even a good diet is no guarantee that your body is doing a good job absorbing nutrients. Sherry Rogers, M.D., of Syracuse, New York, makes the point that "you are what you absorb." Many things can interfere with normal absorption. For example, high-sodium (salt) diets impair calcium absorption, and grains interfere with vitamin D. Sometimes, people have subtle genetic defects that limit vitamin utilization.

Some People Need More Vitamins

The very concept of an RDA may be flawed. In the 1950s, Roger Williams, Ph.D., developed the concept of "biochemical individuality." Williams was one of the most eminent vitamin researchers of the twentieth century.

Biochemical Individuality
Each person is genetically and biochemically unique, meaning we all have varying nutritional requirements in order to maintain health.

Biochemical individuality means that each of us is a nutritional, biochemical, genetic, and anatomical individual. Just as we look different on the outside, each of us requires different amounts of various vitamins. For one person, 100 mg daily of vitamin C might be sufficient for health; for another, 3,000 would be needed.

These differences stem from our genetic individuality, as well as from different conditions when we were in the womb and different conditions as we grew up. As one example, people's stomachs come in all shapes and sizes, and some people produce far more digestive enzymes than do others. The person with good digestion will absorb nutrients better than the person with poor digestion. These differences exist on a very minute level in the body, but they have profound effects on our health and risk of disease.

The bottom line is that everyone needs vitamins and minerals, but different people need different vitamins and minerals in different amounts. One size does not fit all.

Isn't 100 Percent of the RDA Adequate?

The RDA and the DV are extremely conservative estimates of the amounts of vitamins and minerals people need. They are largely designed to prevent the most serious deficiency diseases. The RDA and the DV are not intended as guidelines for optimal intakes for achieving the best health.

The predecessor to today's RDA was designed as a guideline for "practically all healthy persons" by the federal government during World War II. But many prominent nutrition researchers have questioned whether Americans can be considered healthy—and, therefore, whether RDA levels of vitamins are really adequate.

Paul LaChance, Ph.D., of Rutgers University, has pointed out that 30 percent of Americans smoke, and many drink too much alcohol. Others suffer from diabetes, high cholesterol levels, or hypertension. An article in the *Journal of the American Medical Association* recently reported that 45 percent of Americans suffered from at least one chronic condition. "After age 45, most people are not 'healthy' in the strict sense of the word and relatively few qualify as having no chronic or acute problem," LaChance explained in the journal *Nutrition Reviews*.

For example, vitamin B$_6$, folic acid (another B vitamin), and vitamin E are three of the vitamins most important for a healthy heart. A study by Harvard University researchers found that folic acid and vitamin B$_6$ protect against coronary heart disease. However, the most beneficial dose was three or more times the RDA. Similarly, vitamin E seems to offer the most protection to the heart at 400 IU daily—18 times the RDA.

By the way, don't be scared off by a vitamin product that contains 400 percent of the RDA. This amount is 4 times, not 400 times, the RDA.

There's Great Scientific Support for Vitamins

The scientific research supporting the roles of vitamins in health is far better than the research on most drugs. On average, journals publish about 500 to 600 studies a year on vitamin E and about an equal number on vitamin C. In a typical year, more than 5,000 studies are published on vitamins in medical and scientific journals. Over the past thirty-five years, more than 150,000 studies on vitamins have been published, with more than one-third of them published during the 1990s.

If you scrutinize all this research, you'll notice two trends, regardless of whether the studies are on people, animals, or cells. One trend is that higher levels of vitamins and minerals are almost always associated with health. The other is that lower levels of these nutrients are almost always associated with disease.

In the 1940s and 1950s, when a handful of physicians started using vitamins to treat diseases, no one really understood how these nutrients worked. Today, researchers have gained a better understanding of vitamins. For example, vitamin E helps the cardiovascular system by maintaining normal blood vessel flexibility, by reducing the heart-damaging effects of cholesterol, and by blocking the activity of disease-promoting compounds.

Vitamins Protect against Free Radicals

Radicals are hazardous molecules that age us and cause diseases. Bear with us for a few brief paragraphs, because this is about as technical as this book gets: Atoms are the smallest building blocks of everything, living or not. Each atom has electrons circling around its center, much the way planets revolve around the sun. Normally, electrons come in pairs. But when an atom is short one electron (or has one too many), it's called a free radical.

Free Radical

An unpaired electron produced by the body and by pollutants, such as cigarette smoke. Free radicals are involved in all diseases.

The radical is "free" in the sense that it's cruising around aggressively and looking for a partner. If it grabs a replacement electron from an atom that's part of a healthy cell in your body, it damages that cell. Oxygen, which you need to breathe, is the source of most free radicals, so the damage is called "oxidation."

Free radical oxidation is also what makes iron rust and butter turn rancid. Although free radicals are found in air pollution, cigarette smoke, and other nasty compounds, they are also formed when the body burns food for energy. Free radicals are pretty powerful—your body also makes them to kill germs. Too much exposure to sunlight also generates free radicals, which is why sun worshipers tend to have older looking skin.

It helps to think of free radicals as dominoes. One free radical creates another and another and another—until the cascade of free radicals is quenched by an antioxidant vitamin.

Antioxidants to the Rescue

Antioxidants are the flip side of the free radical coin, because they quench (or neutralize) free radicals. Many vitamins and vitaminlike nutrients function as antioxidants, and in doing so, they limit the damage caused by free radicals. Vitamins E and C are antioxidants, as are beta-carotene, lutein, coenzyme Q_{10}, and alpha-lipoic acid.

You Need More than One Antioxidant

Your health will benefit from taking a single antioxidant supplement, such as vitamin E or vitamin C. However, you'll do much better by taking a combination of antioxidants.

Antioxidant
A type of vitamin that donates electrons to stabilize damaging free radicals. Vitamins E and C are two of the most powerful vitamin antioxidants.

Researcher Al L. Tappel, Ph.D., of the University of California, Davis, has shown that a diverse selection of antioxidants may be more important than high doses of just one or two. That doesn't mean you have to swallow handfuls of antioxidant tablets and capsules. For reducing your long-term risk of disease, consider taking an antioxidant "cocktail" containing four to ten different antioxidants. If you're already taking a high-potency multivitamin, you may be getting enough antioxidants.

Lester Packer, Ph.D., has described this antioxidant interaction, or synergism, as the "antioxidant network." Many antioxidants—vitamins E and C, coenzyme Q_{10}, glutathione—work together as a team, helping one another out. Keep in mind, though, that not all vitamins function as antioxidants.

What about Megadosing with Vitamins?

So, what exactly is a megadose of a vitamin? Dietitians, who are generally conservative when it comes to supplements, tend to feel that anything above RDA levels amounts to a megadose. However, the trend in nutrition research is toward developing recommendations that are higher than the current RDAs—that is, more optimal.

A growing number of researchers and physicians believe that vitamin levels roughly three times the RDA are often optimal doses. In an experiment,

Mark Levine, M.D., Ph.D., of the National Institutes of Health, Bethesda, Maryland, found that 200 mg of vitamin C daily—more than twice the RDA—was the ideal intake for young, healthy men. But Levine's study didn't look at women or sick people (about half the population), or people who smoked or were under a lot of stress, so he was reluctant to extrapolate his recommendations to them.

Many others, particularly practicing physicians, have had great success treating patients with so-called megadoses of vitamins. Some of these doctors, such as Hugh Riordan, M.D., of Wichita, Kansas, use laboratory tests to carefully document that patients have low levels of vitamins—and that their improvement follows taking vitamin supplements. Other physicians have developed protocols based on their clinical experiences. Robert Cathcart III, M.D., of Los Altos, California, recommends large amounts of vitamin C (and other vitamins and minerals) to patients with severe infections, ranging from colds and flus to mononucleosis and AIDS.

Why Don't More Doctors Recommend Vitamin Supplements?

Actually, more and more doctors are taking and recommending vitamin supplements. For example, a recent survey of cardiologists found that 44 percent of cardiologists took antioxidants, though only 37 percent also recommended them to patients. Still, physicians do not generally see vitamins as being therapeutic. According to Richard Kunin, M.D., of San Francisco, nutrients are the most dynamic driver of body chemistry.

Other physicians, such as Peter Langsjoen, M.D., a cardiologist in Tyler, Texas, point out that drug companies influence much of a physician's education after medical school. Drug companies are going to market and sell their products, not low-cost natural alternatives. A number of studies have found that physicians tend to prescribe what they hear about the most—just as the average shopper tends to buy the big brand names over the little ones.

Are Excess Vitamins "Expensive Urine"?

There are still some physicians who totally dismiss the use of vitamin supplements, and some have said that excess vitamins lead only to expensive urine. But it's really nothing more than a mean-spirited, irrational argument.

Here's why: If you drink an expensive bottle of wine, you'll also have expensive urine. Ditto for a prime steak—your body will use part of it and turn the rest into expensive stools. Should you then eat and drink the cheapest foods possible? Of course not, you should eat the most nutritious foods possible.

Your body will never absorb 100 percent of any of the food or nutrients you consume. If it did, you'd never have to go to the bathroom. You actually absorb a relatively small portion of what you eat, and it's no different with vitamins. When you take large doses of vitamins, your absorption becomes less efficient—but you'll still absorb more overall than if you took a smaller amount. So, don't pay attention to the critics. After reading this book, you'll probably know more about vitamins and health than they do.

Communicate with Your Physician

Nutritionally oriented physicians usually recommend that patients work with a physician if they want to use vitamins to treat a specific disease. This is good advice. But many people don't take it, perhaps because it's too hard to find a doctor who knows something about vitamins or because their insurance won't reimburse for that doctor's care.

As a consequence, many people end up treating themselves with vitamins, which isn't really all that bad. Vitamins are very safe, and people have a right to treat themselves. (For example, vitamins are safer than aspirin, which many people take to treat headaches without a physician's involvement.) If you have a serious chronic disease, you should, at the very least, let your doctor know you're taking vitamins, even if he or she doesn't believe vitamins have any benefits. You may have to assert yourself and tell your doctor that you intend to take vitamins unless he or she can come up with a good reason why you shouldn't.

It's wise to read up on anything you take, whether it's a vitamin or a prescription drug. While this book is a starting point, there are others that go into more depth about vitamins and how to use them. Some of these books and websites are listed in the Other Books and Resources section toward the end of this book. You can buy many of these books at bookstores and health food stores or borrow them from a public library.

CHAPTER 2

Vitamin A and the Carotenoids

Vitamin A is an essential nutrient found in animal foods, and the carotenoids are found in fruits and vegetables. Beta-carotene, one of the most common carotenoids, can be converted to vitamin A in the body. The carotenoids lutein and lycopene play important roles in health, but the body cannot convert them to vitamin A. Vitamin A has weak antioxidant activity, whereas beta-carotene, lutein, and lycopene are powerful antioxidants with vitaminlike actions.

Vitamin A for Eyes and More

If you've heard that vitamin A is good for the eyes, you heard right. Vitamin A helps convert light to signals that your brain can read, enabling you to see things and distinguish colors. Inadequate intake of vitamin A causes night blindness—a condition in which the eyes have difficulty adjusting to the dark or to bright lights. For this reason, night blindness impairs the vision of drivers. If it takes you more than a minute to adjust your eyes in a darkened theater, you probably have this condition.

Treating night blindness is relatively easy and fast acting. Simply increase your intake of vitamin A–containing foods, such as liver, or take daily supplements—up to 10,000 IU daily. Increasing your intake of fruits and vegetables or taking beta-carotene capsules can help, but these approaches take longer than pure vitamin A.

Vitamin A is essential for the body's production of

epithelial cells, which line most tissues and the skin. Many people find it helpful in skin disorders, such as cystic acne. One recent study found that a form of vitamin A might reverse emphysema in lab rats, but human studies are lacking.

Emphysema
Damage to the wall of the lungs creates large spaces that trap air in this lung disease, causing low blood oxygen levels, shortness of breath, and other problems.

In addition, vitamin A also has hormonelike effects in that it controls the growth and normal differentiation of cells. Differentiation is a normal process that turns new cells into heart cells or lung cells or bone cells. Cancer cells, on the other hand, are *un*differentiated. In other words, vitamin A helps make normal cells.

Vitamin A protects against infection by strengthening the epithelial cell barrier to attacking bacteria and viruses. For years, children in developing nations died from measles, a respiratory disease that has been almost completed eliminated in Western nations. In the mid-1970s, it was discovered that these children were severely deficient in vitamin A and that brief high-dose supplements could cut the death rate from measles by one-third. The preventive dosage is 100,000 IU of vitamin A daily for two days, followed by 100,000 IU one month later.

Some studies have found high doses of vitamin A helpful in other respiratory infections, such as chicken pox and pneumonia. The key is high doses taken for a very short time, such as two days—not long-term, high-dose consumption.

Supplementing with Vitamin A Safely

There is a remote risk of toxicity with vitamin A. That's why recommendations for treating respiratory (lung) infections are high doses for only two days. While the dose—100,000 IU—is very high, it is taken for too short a time to cause side effects (which include hair loss and headaches).

In general, it's quite safe for people to take 10,000

IU of vitamin A daily for many years. Pregnant women, or women who plan to become pregnant, should probably take no more than 8,000 IU of vitamin A daily, because there is a slight risk of birth defects among pregnant women taking very large doses of this vitamin.

Beta-carotene is safe, even at very high doses. In some people, very high doses will turn the skin (particularly hands and feet) a yellow-orange color, but this is not dangerous, and it goes away shortly after supplementation is stopped. Only a small portion of beta-carotene is converted to vitamin A, so you can't create toxic levels of vitamin A by taking a lot of beta-carotene.

Understanding the Carotenoids

The carotenoids are fat-soluble antioxidants that plants produce to protect themselves from the damaging effects of free radicals. Free radicals are one of the basic causes of cancer, heart disease, and other degenerative diseases. Fourteen of the more than 600 carotenoids in nature show up in the blood, indicating that they are absorbed.

Carotenoids
Fat-soluble antioxidants produced by plants that protect cells from free radical damage.

The principal dietary carotenoids appear to be beta-carotene (found in carrots), alpha-carotene (also found in carrots), lutein (found in kale, broccoli, and spinach), and lycopene (found in tomatoes). Other important—though minor—carotenoids are zeaxanthin and cryptoxanthin. When we eat foods containing carotenoids, we benefit from their antioxidant properties.

For example, in addition to being a source of vitamin A, beta-carotene quenches a type of free radical called "singlet oxygen." Several studies have reported that beta-carotene increases lung capacity—basically the amount of oxygen you can breathe in and out. The more oxygen you can take in with a single breath, the healthier you are. This is because all of our cells need adequate oxygen to do their jobs well. Lung capacity generally decreases with age.

Beta-carotene Research Results

Two studies found that beta-carotene slightly increased the risk of lung cancer among current smokers, particularly if they also drank alcohol. But these studies used synthetic beta-carotene. The synthetic form does not contain the powerful antioxidant found in natural beta-carotene supplements, which comes from *Dunaliella salina* algae. Even so, one of these studies found that former smokers taking beta-carotene had a lower risk of developing lung cancer.

Many studies have reported that beta-carotene taken with other antioxidants, such as vitamin E and selenium, is good for health. Beta-carotene seems to work best as part of an antioxidant team rather than by itself. Taking supplements containing "mixed carotenoids" and additional antioxidant vitamins as opposed to beta-carotene alone is recommended.

Several studies have found that a combination of beta-carotene supplements (taken orally) and conventional sunscreens (applied to the skin) work better than sunscreens alone. In a sense, beta-carotene helps provide inside-out protection against the ultraviolet (UV) radiation in sunlight. It most likely works by improving the skin's natural and internal defenses against UV damage.

Carotenoids for Eye and Prostate Health

The macula is the center of the eye's retina, acting kind of like a theater screen, and its premature breakdown is the leading cause of blindness among Americans over age sixty-five. Two carotenoids, lutein and zeaxanthin, seem to help preserve the macula. Together, they form the yellowish macular pigment that filters out damaging ultraviolet light and protects lipid-rich membranes from free radical damage.

A study published in *The Journal of the American Medical Association* (*JAMA*) found that people who eat foods rich in lutein—particularly kale and spinach—were less likely to develop macular degeneration. Studies have reported that consuming lutein-rich foods or supplements increases the thickness of the macular pigment. Lutein supplements may not reverse macular degeneration, but researchers believe it can slow the progression of this disease.

Zeaxanthin is also important to the macula, but it appears that the body can convert some lutein to zeaxanthin. There is evidence that lutein and zeaxanthin (both found in the eye lens) may also help slow the development of cataracts, but it's unclear whether these two carotenoids could actually reverse cataracts.

Recent studies on lutein and zeaxanthin have found that supplements increase the thickness of the macular pigment and, consequently, should reduce the long-term risk of macular degeneration. These nutrients work, in part, like polarizing sunglasses—they filter out stray light particles so they do not damage the eye.

Lycopene May Benefit the Prostate Gland

Some carotenoids, especially lycopene and beta-carotene, appear to benefit the prostate. In a study in the *Journal of the National Cancer Institute,* Edward Giovannucci, M.D., of Harvard University, reported that men eating large amounts of tomato sauce (more than ten servings weekly) were 45 percent less likely to develop prostate cancer. Raw tomatoes provided some benefit, but tomato juice didn't help at all.

Cooking tomatoes (for example, for spaghetti or pizza sauces) breaks down the cell walls containing lycopene, making more of this nutrient available for digestion and absorption. Such sauces are also made with olive oil, which aids lycopene absorption (because it is fat-soluble). Raw tomatoes are typically eaten with either salad dressing or meat, so the oil or fat in these foods aids absorption. Tomato juice is not cooked; nor does it contain additional oil.

Another Harvard University study found that, among men not eating fruits and vegetables, beta-carotene supplements reduced the risk of prostate cancer by one-third. High dietary intakes of lutein and zeaxanthin have also been associated with reduced prostate cancer risk.

CHAPTER 3

THE B-VITAMIN COMPLEX

Together, the eleven B vitamins influence many aspects of health. For example, the B vitamins affect energy levels, mood, behavior, and risk of degenerative diseases, including heart disease and cancer. This chapter covers some of the ways B vitamins can improve your health.

Stress Relief and Improved Mood

The B vitamins have long been regarded as anti-stress vitamins. They are important for normal nerve and brain function, so inadequate levels of them interfere with the nervous system. According to David Benton, Ph.D., a researcher and professor at the University of Wales Swansea, the first signs of vitamin deficiencies are psychological problems. Among these are irritability, anger, and difficulty dealing with pressures at home or work.

To help combat stress, consider taking a B-complex supplement. Look on the label to make sure that it contains 10 mg of vitamin B_1, also known as thiamine—this is a clue to the relative amounts of the other B vitamins in the supplement. If you don't sense any improvement after thirty days, either triple the dose or buy a B-complex supplement with 25 mg of vitamin B_1.

Vitamin B_1 can also improve mood. Benton gave healthy students either a high-potency multivitamin (containing ten times the RDA of most vitamins) or a placebo (dummy pill) for a year. When he reevaluated the mood of the students, Benton found that the multivitamin group described themselves as more agreeable, and the women said their moods had improved significantly, according to his article in *Biological Psychology/Pharmacopsychology.*

While all of the vitamins seemed to help, vitamin B_1 stood out among the others. This may be because popular high-carbohydrate diets reduce vitamin B_1 activity. In a follow-up study that Benton conducted, female university students taking vitamin B_1 described themselves as more clearheaded, self-composed, and energetic after two months of supplementation. They also had faster reaction times.

Another B vitamin, folic acid, seems to improve mood, too. Low levels of this vitamin have been found in a significant percentage of adults suffering from depression. Supplementing with therapeutic amounts of folic acid has improved depression in many patients, according to recent research.

Lowering Cholesterol with Niacin

The niacin form of vitamin B_3 has been known since 1955 to lower cholesterol levels, which results in decreased heart disease risk. This was discovered by Abram Hoffer, M.D., Ph.D., one of the pioneers in the medical use of vitamins. Other forms of vitamin B_3, such as niacinamide, do not have this cholesterol-lowering effect.

Before you take niacin, be aware of its principal side effect. After taking it, you will have a body-wide flushing, or tingling, sensation. Your skin will turn beet red and you'll feel itchy all over. This reaction can be a little unsettling, but it is not harmful. The warm, flushing sensation (which some people even like) passes after about an hour.

If you continually take niacin three times a day, the flushing reaction will lessen and eventually stop. Hoffer recommends taking 500 mg of niacin three times daily. Vitamin C supplements—1,000 mg daily—can also sometimes reduce blood cholesterol levels, without flushing.

Vitamin B₃ for Schizophrenia

Schizophrenia is a mental disorder characterized by delusions (such as extreme paranoia) and hallucinations (seeing or hearing things that aren't there); it is not the same as split personality. In the early 1950s, Abram Hoffer, M.D., Ph.D., and Humphry Osmond, M.D., theorized that some types of schizophrenics were producing a hallucinogen in their own bodies. The hallucinogen was an oxidized form of adrenaline.

Based on their knowledge of biochemistry, these researchers believed that high doses of vitamin B_3 (either niacin or niacinamide) and vitamin C would neutralize this hallucinogen. They turned out to be right. The researchers published the first double-blind trial in the field of psychiatry in the *Bulletin of the Menninger Clinic*.

Hoffer usually gives schizophrenic patients 3,000 mg of vitamin B_3 and 1,000–3,000 mg of vitamin C daily. He has pointed out that patients with a recent onset of schizophrenia respond better to vitamin therapy than do patients who have suffered from schizophrenia for a very long time. Also, some schizophrenic patients respond better to high doses of vitamin B_6 and zinc, an essential dietary mineral.

Vitamins for Carpal Tunnel Syndrome Relief

Carpal tunnel syndrome is characterized by extreme pain or numbness in the wrist and hand. It is caused by the stress of a repetitive hand motion. Supermarket cashiers, typists, and factory workers are prone to it.

Some thirty years ago, John Ellis, M.D., of Mount Pleasant, Texas, found that vitamin B_6 could help patients with carpal tunnel syndrome. He found that patients with this disorder had low levels of vitamin B_6 and that taking 100 mg daily would restore normal levels after ninety days. Other researchers have also found strong associations between low vitamin B_6 levels and carpal tunnel syndrome. It's likely that the repetitive stress increases vitamin B_6 requirements.

It's unusual, however, for a person to be deficient in just one nutrient, and the B vitamins work together as a family of related nutrients. A better regimen for carpal tunnel might be 100 mg of vitamin B_6, plus a B-complex supplement containing all members of this family.

Normalizing Homocysteine Levels

Homocysteine is a byproduct of protein found in the blood. High blood levels of homocysteine cause free radical damage to blood vessel walls and set the stage for cholesterol deposits. Eventually, these deposits, or "plaques," can obstruct blood flow, increasing the risk of coronary heart disease.

Unlike cholesterol, homocysteine in not found in foods. Homocysteine levels rise when a person consumes too much protein (especially red meat) relative to B vitamins. A number of B vitamins are involved in breaking down homocysteine or recycling it back to protein. Folic acid appears to be the most important of these, but vitamins B_6 and B_{12} are also involved.

Homocysteine
An amino acid found in the blood and a byproduct of protein metabolism. At high levels, it damages blood vessel walls, increasing the risk of heart disease.

Research has also pointed to a likely relationship between elevated homocysteine levels, B vitamins, and the risk of Alzheimer's disease. Low blood levels of vitamin B_{12} and/or folic acid, as well as elevated homocysteine levels, greatly increase one's risk of developing the disease, according to recent studies. Folic acid supplementation can also reduce the risk of neural tube defects (like spina bifida) in babies when taken by the mother prior to conception and during pregnancy.

Quick and relatively inexpensive ways to test homocysteine levels are now available. In general, the lower the homocysteine level, the better; a level of less than 6 micromoles per liter of blood is ideal. Heart disease risk increases with the level, and more than 13 micromoles per liter is considered very dangerous. Supplements of 400 mcg of folic acid daily should normalize elevated homocysteine levels. Again, it may be best to take this amount as part of a B-complex supplement.

Multiple Sclerosis and Vitamin B$_{12}$

Multiple sclerosis, or MS, is characterized by damage to the sheaths that protect neurons of the central nervous system. Muscle weakness, visual impairment, lack of coordination, and other problems can result. The cause of the disease and satisfactory treatment are unknown.

A number of studies have found that people with MS are consistently deficient in vitamin B$_{12}$. Low levels of folic acid may also be a problem, as these two vitamins work hand in hand.

Multiple Sclerosis
A disease in which the protective coatings around neurons in the central nervous system deteriorate, slowing and short-circuiting nerve impulse conduction.

Many people have trouble absorbing B$_{12}$ through the gut. Injections of B$_{12}$ administered by a doctor can get around this problem. So can sublingual tablets, which are small and meant to dissolve under the tongue (where absorption is very efficient).

More B-Vitamin Benefits

If you have arthritis, listen up. Years ago, doctors found that they could ease symptoms of rheumatoid arthritis by giving one of the B vitamins, then ease symptoms some more by giving another B vitamin. It might be faster and more effective to simply take a high-potency B-complex supplement, rather than trying the B vitamins one by one.

One study, reported in the *Journal of the American College of Nutrition*, found that daily supplements of folic acid (6,400 mcg) and vitamin B_{12} (20 mcg) relieved symptoms of osteoarthritis of the hands. A more recent study, in the German journal *Schmerz*, described the analgesic (pain-relieving) properties of vitamins B_1, B_2, and B_{12}. The researcher noted that the combination of these vitamins is more effective than any of them individually.

Two recent studies showed that vitamin B_2 may reduce the frequency of migraine headaches. About two-thirds of migraine patients given 400 mg of B_2 daily for at least three months improved significantly. Only a small number in a placebo group improved. (Vitamin B_2 can make urine bright yellow, but this is its natural color and not harmful.)

Women experiencing premenstrual syndrome, or PMS, might find relief with B vitamins as well. PMS is often caused by excess estrogen, a female hormone. Two B vitamins, choline and inositol, help convert estrogen into estriol, a form of the hormone that doesn't seem to cause problems. In addition, vitamin B_6 is a diuretic and can prevent water retention before your period. Again, if you take B_6 (50–100 mg daily), add a B-complex supplement.

CHAPTER 4

VITAMIN C

Vitamin C is abundant in fruits and vegetables, but most people do not eat as many of these foods as they should. Have you eaten your three to five (or, as some organizations recommend, five to nine) servings of fruits and vegetables today? Probably not. For this reason alone, you could likely benefit from vitamin C supplements.

The Vitamin C and Cold Connection

In 1970, Nobel laureate Linus Pauling, Ph.D., recommended large doses of vitamin C in his book *Vitamin C and the Common Cold.* According to scientific studies published since then, Pauling was on to something. Vitamin C can reduce the symptoms and the length of colds and flu. There's no evidence suggesting that it prevents them, though; washing your hands after contact with an infected person is probably more preventive.

There have been dozens of scientific studies investigating vitamin C's effects on the common cold. Harri Hemilä, Ph.D., a researcher at the University of Helsinki, Finland, analyzed these studies as a group and found that taking 2–6 g (2,000–6,000 mg) of vitamin C daily, beginning at the first symptoms of a cold, cut the length and severity of the cold by about 30 percent. The minimum effective dose appeared to be 1 g (1,000 mg) daily. Another recent review also found that taking relatively high doses of vitamin C at a cold's onset does appear reduce symptom duration, at least modestly.

Vitamin C works by enhancing your immune system's ability to fight infections. It increases the activity of white blood cells, T cells, and antibodies—all of which help kill bacteria and viruses. It also cleans up excess free radicals, which your body produces to fight bacteria and viruses.

Robert Cathcart III, M.D., of Los Altos, California, has for years recommended high doses of vitamin C to patients with much more serious infections, including mononucleosis and HIV/AIDS. Cathcart has used extremely high doses—from 25–100 grams daily—to treat these severe infections.

Vitamin C and Cancer

In the 1970s, Ewan Cameron, M.D., of Scotland, treated terminal cancer patients with large doses of vitamin C. In general, they lived longer than did patients not given vitamin C. A small number of patients were considered "cured." Over the past ten years, Abram Hoffer, M.D., Ph.D., of Victoria, Canada, has treated terminal cancer patients with large doses of vitamin C combined with other vitamins and minerals. About one-third of his earliest patients, who were judged terminal, have lived more than ten years and are considered, by conventional criteria, to be "cured."

Some types of cancer respond better than others to vitamin C. For example, women with reproductive cancers, such as breast cancer, respond to vitamin therapy much better than people with lung cancer. Hoffer's cancer regimen includes the following nutrients on a daily basis; the doses may vary from patient to patient.

Vitamin C	12 grams or more
Coenzyme Q_{10}	300 mg
Vitamin B_3	500 mg–3 grams
Vitamin B_6	250 mg for some (not all) patients
Folic acid	5–10 mg (not mcg)
Other B vitamins	25 to 50 times the RDA

Vitamin E	800 IU in the "succinate" form
Carotenoids	25,000–50,000 IU
Selenium	200–600 mcg
Zinc	220 mg (or 59 mg zinc citrate)

Of course, if you have cancer, it's best to work with a physician instead of treating yourself. If you have already had surgery, chemotherapy, or radiation, these supplements can enhance your immune system so your body does a better job of fighting recurrent cancer.

Vitamin C and Rheumatism

Vitamin C can protect against arthritis and rheumatism, though it likely works best in combination with B-complex vitamins. In rheumatism and rheumatoid arthritis, weak capillaries (our tiniest blood vessels) leak blood cells into the joints. The immune system responds as if these blood cells were invading bacteria, triggering a painful inflammatory response.

Rheumatism
A painful disorder of the body's supporting structures, including bones, joints, and muscles. Rheumatoid arthritis involves inflamed joints.

Supplemental vitamin C strengthens capillary walls, as do antioxidant flavonoids (vitaminlike nutrients found in fruits and vegetables). In this way, they prevent leakage from blood vessels and the resulting inflammatory response. Vitamin C is also essential for the body's manufacture of collagen, a protein needed to form the soft tissue in bone joints and the skin.

In a recent issue of the French medical journal *Revue Du Rhumatisme,* Jean Léone, M.D., of the Robert Debré Teaching Hospital in Reims, describes how two patients with rheumatism were actually suffering from scurvy (rheumatism was a symptom of scurvy). Scurvy is a severe vitamin C deficiency disease characterized by bleeding gums and other abnormal bleeding, such as wounds that do not heal.

(The bleeding is caused by weak capillary walls.) Léone's patients recovered after he gave them 1,000 mg of vitamin C daily for ten days.

Additional Potential Benefits

In a study directed by Allen Taylor, Ph.D., of Tufts University, Boston, vitamin C supplements dramatically reduced the risk of developing cataracts. A cataract is the clouding of the eye's lens, which impairs vision. It can be caused by excessive exposure to UV sunlight, medications, injury, and disease complications. While cataracts are easily corrected with surgery (in which the lens is removed and replaced by a plastic one), it's always best to avoid surgery. Also, cataracts may be a sign of other looming health problems.

In Taylor's study, he found that women who took at least 400 mg of vitamin C supplements daily—for more than ten years—were about 80 percent less likely to develop cataracts. Dietary vitamin C didn't offer this protection. The association between higher blood levels of vitamin C and decreased cataract risk has been supported by more recent research, too.

Cataract
Clouding over of the normally transparent eye lens, impairing vision. It is often associated with aging and diabetes.

Vitamin C may even help allergies because it has a slight antihistaminic effect, like many allergy medications. During allergic reactions, the body releases a compound called histamine, which makes you red and itchy. Vitamin C does not have any of the negative side effects associated with antihistamine drugs. For example, it will not make you drowsy. It is also essential for normal immune function, and it likely corrects some of the immune defects involved in allergies.

Vitamin C might reduce the risk of gallbladder disease. Your gallbladder stores bile, a substance that helps digest fats. Gallstones are rich in cholesterol, and vitamin C limits their formation by activating an enzyme that breaks cholesterol down into bile acids. An estimated 20 million Americans suffer from gallstones, and the typical person with gallbladder disorders is an overweight, middle-aged woman.

Joel A. Simon, M.D., of the University of California, San Francisco, found that among 2,744 women, those consuming large amounts of vitamin C—particularly from supplements—had a 26 percent lower risk of developing gallbladder disease (of all types) and a 23 percent lower risk of having their gallbladders removed, compared with women consuming little vitamin C.

More recent research, based on data from the Third National Health and Nutrition Examination Survey, supports these findings. This time, vitamin C supplements on their own were associated with a 34 percent lower prevalence of gallstones in women. Total vitamin C intake was linked to a 39 percent lower risk among women. Vitamin C did not influence gallstone risk among men.

Taking Vitamin C Supplements

Most people can benefit from 1,000–2,000 mg of vitamin C daily. Even 500 mg is better than nothing. If you're willing to take higher dosages, follow Cathcart's concept of adjusting the dose to "bowel tolerance." He recommends increasing your vitamin C dose (divided up several times daily) until your stools become loose, and then lowering the dose slightly.

Cathcart has found that the sicker a person is, the more vitamin C he or she can tolerate without diarrhea. For example, if you get an average cold, your vitamin C tolerance may increase to 10 grams a day. If you get a very bad cold, your vitamin C tolerance may increase to 25 grams a day. As you start to get better, your vitamin C requirements will decrease. For example, when you're in good health, you may be able to tolerate only 1–3 grams of vitamin C a day.

For most people, the ideal dose of vitamin C is just under the amount that causes loose stools and diarrhea. Divide your dosage so you take a little of it two to four times per day. This increases absorption and decreases the likelihood of developing diarrhea.

Some evidence suggests that many people don't get enough vitamin C. Early signs of a deficiency include tiredness and irritability; advanced signs include bleeding gums, bruising, sores that take a long time to heal, frequent colds, and extreme fatigue. Vitamin C is considered very safe for nearly everyone in the general population at levels up to 2 grams daily, according to The Food and Nutrition Board of the Institute of Medicine of the United States and Canada. One study, published in 1998, reported that 500 mg of vitamin C damaged DNA, but the subsequent experiments by the researchers found just the opposite: That vitamin C protected DNA.

CHAPTER 5

VITAMINS D AND K FOR HEALTHY BONES

It's often assumed that people get adequate quantities of vitamin D, but low intake may be fairly common. The vitamin works with calcium, an essential mineral, to help build strong bones and teeth. Thus, it plays an important role in preventing osteoporosis, the disease in which bones become porous, fragile, and susceptible to fracture.

The Calcium Helper

You probably already know that calcium is important for building and maintaining strong bones. But calcium needs vitamin D to do its job. That's because vitamin D enhances the absorption of calcium.

Research results have shown that treating vitamin D deficiency results in a significant reduction of hip fractures in patients with osteoporosis. In a separate study, reported in the *New England Journal of Medicine,* a combination of calcium (500 mg daily) and vitamin D (700 IU daily) increased bone density in several hundred elderly men and women.

Osteoporosis and osteoarthritis are not the same problem, but vitamin D may play a role in both. In one study, Timothy E. McAlindon, M.D., of the Boston University Arthritis Center, found that patients were more likely to have osteoarthritis of the knees if they did not consume 400 IU of vitamin D daily. Vitamin D has hormonelike roles in the body, so it probably influences the growth of cells involved in healthy joints.

"D" for Deficiency

Children might get enough vitamin D from milk, but not all milk is fortified with vitamin D and many adults don't drink much milk. Your body can make its own vitamin D with the sun's help. Spending at least fifteen minutes in the sun at least three or four times each week is considered adequate. Yet many people with office jobs and elderly people restricted to their homes don't get outside much or may face cloudy weather when they do.

Elderly, frail people are especially susceptible to vitamin D deficiency. In a study of 290 patients, Melissa K. Thomas, M.D., Ph.D., of Massachusetts General Hospital, Boston, found that 164 patients over age sixty-five were deficient in vitamin D, and 22 percent were severely deficient. Even many younger subjects turned out to be deficient in vitamin D. Thomas found that 42 percent of men and women, ranging from the late thirties to the late fifties in age, were low in vitamin D.

Supplementation can ensure that you get enough vitamin D. Very high doses for extended periods can be toxic, but getting 400–800 IU daily is safe for adults. (The RDA is 400 IU daily.) Some experts recommend 800 IU daily for those over age sixty-five and 400 IU daily for younger people.

And What about Vitamin K?

Vitamin K, also called phylloquinone, is a fat-soluble vitamin needed to help blood platelet cells clot after a cut or incision. Without vitamin K, you would bleed to death from the slightest scratch. It is also essential for brain development. According to M. J. Shearer, Ph.D., of St. Thomas's Hospital, London, babies who were deficient in this vitamin during the first six months of their lives risk permanent brain damage or death.

Recent research has emphasized the role of vitamin K in bone formation. Osteocalcin is one of the proteins involved in bone development. To build bone, osteocalcin must be loaded by chemical structures known as carboxyl groups. Your body uses vitamin K to help attach these carboxyl groups to osteocalcin. In a study of nine healthy women at Tufts University, Boston, James A. Sadlowski, Ph.D., found that vitamin K supplements increased the attachment of carboxyl groups to osteocalcin, setting the stage for bone formation.

Sadlowski's study used 420 mcg of vitamin K daily, which is about four times the RDA. Some study findings suggest that vitamin K intakes much higher than current recommendations improve bone health. In addition, researchers found that low vitamin K intake may increase hip fracture risk in women, based on results from the Nurses' Health Study cohort. This has led some experts to suggest that vitamin K requirements be reassessed.

According to an article in the *Journal of Nutrition*, the vitamin K content of most foods is low. Leafy green vegetables are excellent dietary sources. However, absorption of vitamin K from foods is poor, so supplements may be beneficial. If you take a multivitamin, make sure there's some vitamin K in it.

CHAPTER 6

VITAMIN E FOR HEART AND MIND

Years ago, doctors dismissed vitamin E as the "sex vitamin" and a "cure in search of a disease." Yet time has been on this amazing vitamin's side. Studies have found that vitamin E supplements can reduce your risk of coronary heart disease and stroke. It can slow the progression of Alzheimer's disease and maybe prevent it. It can even help your immune system.

Vitamin E and Heart Health

In the 1940s, Evan Shute, M.D., and his brother Wilfrid Shute, M.D., of Canada, pioneered the use of vitamin E supplements in the prevention and treatment of coronary heart disease. Even *Time* magazine wrote about their work in 1946. But most doctors believed vitamins cured only vitamin-deficiency diseases, not conditions like heart disease. So while the Shutes went on to treat tens of thousands of patients with vitamin E over the years, most doctors felt vitamin E was worthless.

Meanwhile, researchers conducted basic research on vitamin E and found it to be a powerful antioxidant and the body's principal fat-soluble antioxidant. In the early 1990s, researchers at Harvard University reported that supplements of vitamin E greatly reduced the risk of heart disease and heart attacks. A 1996 study published in the British journal *Lancet* showed that vitamin E supplements—400–800 IU daily—reduced the incidence of heart attack by 77 percent. Since then, vitamin E has practically become a standard part of mainstream medicine. Many physicians take vitamin E and recommend it to their patients. An analysis of the five largest trials investigating vitamin E for heart health, published in the journal *Current Opinion in Lipidology* in 2001, concluded that alpha-tocopherol (the most common form of vitamin E) was beneficial in patients with preexisting heart disease. (The one study showing no benefit was criticized for design flaws.)

Vitamin E's antioxidant power helps explain how it keeps cholesterol from damaging your blood vessels. Low-density lipoprotein, the so-called "bad" form of cholesterol commonly referred to as LDL, is actually needed to transport vitamin E and the carotenoids through the bloodstream. When there is insufficient vitamin E in the LDL, that LDL is prone to oxidation, or free radical damage.

LDL
Low-density lipoprotein, or LDL, transports proteins, triglycerides (fats), cholesterol, and fat-soluble vitamins through the blood to body cells.

Oxidized LDL builds up on blood vessel walls over time, limiting normal blood flow. In studies with people, Ishwarlal Jialal, M.D., of the University of Texas Southwestern Medical Center, Dallas, found that vitamin E supplements protect LDL from oxidation, thus preventing LDL deposits in blood vessels and reducing the risk of coronary heart disease.

Vitamin E can benefit even those eating a diet high in fat, but eating healthfully is best, of course. In a study described in the *Journal of the American Medical Association,* Gary D. Plotnick, M.D., of the University of Maryland School of Medicine, Baltimore, found that high-fat foods prevent blood vessels from relaxing. The long-term effect is to increase blood pressure and the risk of heart disease. When Plotnick gave his subjects (men and women) 800 IU of vitamin E and 1,000 mg of vitamin C, their blood vessels behaved normally after eating a high-fat, high-carbohydrate meal.

Vitamin E and Reproductive Health

When vitamin E was discovered in 1922, it was called the "fertility vitamin" because rodents deficient in vitamin E became sterile. Being infertile, of course, is different from being impotent. Still, people started referring to vitamin E as the sex vitamin.

Some men with impotency may improve with vitamin E, though the improvement won't happen overnight. This is because impotence is often related to cardiovascular disease. In impotency, the blood vessels of the penis become as damaged as those of the heart. So anything that improves cardiovascular disease—including vitamin E—might also help in impotency.

Vitamin E improves blood flow to all tissues, including those in the penis. Every condition improves with better blood flow. However, if you are impotent because of psychological reasons, like performance anxiety, vitamin E probably won't help.

Several studies, published in *Fertility and Sterility*, have reported that infertile men have high levels of free radicals and low levels of antioxidants in their semen. For this reason, many urologists recommend vitamin E and other antioxidants to infertile men. It takes at least three months for vitamins to have an effect, mainly because it takes that long for sperm to mature. Infertile couples should both take supplemental vitamin E and a high-potency multivitamin for several months before trying to conceive.

More Good News

The list of vitamin E benefits doesn't end with reproductive and heart health. Researchers have found that this incredible vitamin seems to slow the progression of Alzheimer's disease. This debilitating disease affects about 20 million people in the world, robbing them of healthy minds. There is currently no cure for Alzheimer's disease.

Mary Sano, Ph.D., of Columbia University's College of Physicians and Surgeons, New York, and her colleagues found that 2,000 IU of vitamin E (a very large dose) given to severe Alzheimer's patients for two years delayed the progression of end-stage Alzheimer's disease by eight months compared with the placebo group. After Sano's study was published in the *New England Journal of Medicine*, the American Psychiatric Association recommended that Alzheimer's patients receive vitamin E. Since then, the American Academy of Neurology and the Alzheimer's Association have officially encouraged physicians to use 1,000 IU of vitamin E, twice daily, to slow the progression of Alzheimer's disease.

There are a couple of reasons that vitamin E may slow Alzheimer's disease—and possibly even prevent or delay its onset. This nutrient is essential for normal functioning of cell membranes, or walls. These cell membranes have doors that allow vitamins and other nutrients in and waste products out. These membranes harden with age, but vitamin E seems to keep them younger and suppler. In addition, vitamin E limits free radical damage to brain cells, and high levels of free radicals are thought to be a major cause of Alzheimer's disease.

Alzheimer's Disease
A degenerative brain disease caused by neuron dysfunction and death that causes problems with memory, feelings, thinking, and behavior.

Several studies show that vitamin E can enhance resistance to infection. This is particularly important for older folks, because the immune system declines with age. In a study at Tufts University, Boston, researchers found that 200 IU of vitamin E daily improved immune responsiveness significantly, meaning that the immune system would be more likely to respond to infection during a bacterial attack. Subjects taking vitamin E had 30 percent fewer infections, too. Other studies have found that vitamin E (as well as the mineral selenium) can prevent dangerous mutations in the Coxsackie virus, which infects some 20 million Americans a year, causing sore throats and coldlike symptoms.

If you feel wiped out after a workout, consider upping your vitamin E intake. Your body's cells produce free radicals as a byproduct of normal activities, called metabolism. When you exercise, you speed up the process and generate more free radicals. So ironically, excessive exercise is bad. The solution is not to become a couch potato, but to take vitamin E and other antioxidants.

These vitamins prevent DNA (genetic) damage and oxidation of cell fats caused by overexercise. According to Lester Packer, Ph.D., a researcher at the University of California, Berkeley, and one of the foremost authorities on antioxidants, vitamin E can probably reduce exercise-induced fatigue. Quicker recovery from fatigue can improve exercise performance.

Taking Vitamin E

As Americans, our vitamin E requirements are very high, in part, because we eat large quantities of refined oils (for example, in salad dressing, French fries, and many other foods). These oils are very prone to oxidation, and vitamin E protects against their oxidation, in and out of the body. So the more fats you eat, the higher your vitamin E needs are.

Most experts seem to have settled on 400 IU of vitamin E daily as the best dose for heart health support and other benefits. Some studies have shown that levels as low as 100 IU provide some benefit and that higher doses (800 IU–1,200 IU) are safe, though probably unnecessary. It's virtually impossible to get 400 IU of vitamin E from diet alone. It's been estimated that you'd have to eat 1,000 almonds to get 400 IU of vitamin E—and all those almonds would contain 8,000 calories and more than a pound of fat.

Natural vitamin E (most of which comes from soybeans) is better for you than the synthetic form. Over the years, studies have found that natural vitamin E is about 36 percent more biologically active than the synthetic form. A recent study by Graham W. Burton,

Ph.D., of Canada's National Research Council, found that natural vitamin E was absorbed twice as efficiently as the synthetic form.

d-alpha tocopherol
The form of natural vitamin E most abundant in our bodies and most often used in vitamin supplements. It supports reproduction and promotes good health.

It's easy to distinguish between synthetic and natural forms of vitamin E with a little detective work. Synthetic vitamin E will be identified by its chemical name, "dl-alpha tocopherol" or "dl-alpha tocopheryl acetate" on the nutrition facts panel of supplement bottle labels. In contrast, natural vitamin E is called "d-alpha tocopherol," "d-alpha tocopheryl acetate," or "d-alpha tocopheryl succinate." In other words, "dl" signifies synthetic and "d" denotes natural vitamin E.

There's a simple way to remember the difference. The "d" means that it is delicious to your body; conversely, your body doesn't like the "dl" (or synthetic) form as much. There are various vitamin E compounds, but the key is to look for the "d," which indicates natural.

Some experts believe that a "full-spectrum" vitamin E supplement is even better than d-alpha tocopherol alone. Unlike most vitamins, vitamin E has eight different forms, known as stereoisomers. Alpha-tocopherol is the most well known. The other forms are also important to health in ways that researchers are just beginning to understand. This is why Andreas Papas, Ph.D., one of today's foremost vitamin E experts, recommends that people seek out a supplement containing all eight forms of vitamin E, often listed on labels as "mixed tocotrienols" and "mixed tocopherols." Together, the thinking goes, the eight forms of vitamin E work as a team to keep us healthy. (Again, look for the natural form.)

Vitamin E for Diabetes

People with diabetes taking insulin or hypoglycemic

drugs should start taking vitamins at a low dose and gradually increase the dose, unless their physician asks them to take higher doses sooner. Because most vitamins are involved in converting blood sugar, or glucose, to energy, vitamins may speed up this process and lower glucose levels. So you have to exercise a little caution at first.

The good news is that anyone with diabetes can benefit from vitamin supplementation. Glucose generates large numbers of free radicals, and this gets out of hand in diabetic people because they have high glucose levels. These free radicals oxidize cholesterol and damage blood vessel walls; this is one reason why people with diabetes have an above-average risk of developing cardiovascular diseases.

Vitamin E and a vitaminlike antioxidant, alpha-lipoic acid, help control these excess free radicals and reduce the damage. Alpha-lipoic acid (300–600 mg daily for diabetes) may also lower glucose levels by 10 to 30 percent, but the glucose levels also stabilize, which is better for controlling diabetes. Other vitamins, such as vitamin C and the B-complex vitamins, also help control diabetes and diabetic complications.

Vitamin E and Heart Disease Patients

Even people who already have heart disease can benefit from boosting vitamin E intake. As mentioned earlier, authors of a recent analysis of large-scale trials of vitamin E supplementation found that four out of the five supported a benefit for vitamin E supplementation in patients who already had heart disease. (The fifth study was criticized for design flaws.) Subjects taking vitamin E (the alpha-tocopherol form) supplements in these studies had a dramatically reduced risk of nonfatal heart attack.

Substantial research shows that vitamin E and other antioxidant vitamins can reduce the risk of complications from heart surgery. Heart surgery is a major stress, and about 3 percent of people undergoing bypass surgery do not survive. It's crucial for heart disease patients to check with their doctors before supplementing with vitamin E, however. Large doses of vitamin E could potentially thin the blood too much in patients who already take prescription blood thinners like Coumadin.

During bypass surgery, blood flow is stopped so doctors can graft new arteries. When blood flow is replenished, large numbers of free radicals are generated, and these radicals can damage the heart. Some heart surgeons give their patients vitamin E supplements before surgery to limit this damage.

CHAPTER 7

WHAT MINERALS CAN DO FOR YOUR HEALTH

By now, you surely realize that vitamins offer amazing health benefits, but the story doesn't end there. There's another group of micronutrients that deserves your attention. This group is made up of essential minerals. They're referred to as essential because the body needs them to function correctly and we must get them from the diet; the body can't make them on its own. Minerals make up only about 4 percent of one's total body weight, but their importance is weighty indeed.

Minerals Defined

As we mentioned earlier, minerals are elements, which means that they cannot be broken down into simpler substances. Unlike vitamins, which come from living organisms, minerals come from nonliving matter. This is why we refer to minerals as inorganic, or nonliving.

Minerals are usually ingested as compounds (in combination with other minerals or organic compounds) as opposed to solitary elements, whether they be in food or supplement form. Minerals must be freed from their compounds during digestion so they can be absorbed and used by the body.

There are two groups of minerals that everyone needs: macrominerals (or major minerals) and microminerals (often called trace minerals). Macrominerals are considered the major minerals because they make up more body weight than the microminerals. The body requires each macromineral in an amount greater than 100 milligrams per day from diet and supplement intake. Calcium, magnesium, chloride, sodium, potassium, phosphorus, and sulfur are macrominerals.

The remaining essential minerals—iron, zinc, selenium, manganese, chromium, cobalt, molybdenum, iodine, fluorine, and copper—are microminerals. These are usually required in amounts less than 100 milligrams per day—but that doesn't mean that they are any less crucial for good health. Other trace minerals—silicon and vanadium, for example—are essential in animals and thought to be essential in humans, too.

Macro- and Microminerals

Macrominerals are minerals that the body needs in amounts greater than 100 milligrams each day. Microminerals are those that the body requires in smaller amounts.

The Myriad Roles of Minerals

Minerals play an impressive array of roles in the body. Calcium, for one, helps make bones and teeth hard, regulates hormones, and is involved in muscle contractions, blood clotting, and more. Minerals regulate many body processes and are needed for brain function, fluid regulation, acid-base balance, bone growth, enzyme action, carrying oxygen in the blood, making fatty acids, digesting protein, and so on.

Some minerals act as electrolytes, which are salts found in body fluids that maintain electrical neutrality. Electrolytes called cations have a positive electrical charge, while anions are negatively charged. A proper ratio of cations to anions is needed to keep the body in balance at all times.

Like vitamins, many minerals are finally gaining attention for their incredible antioxidant powers. As you'll remember from earlier chapters, antioxidants neutralize pesky free radicals before they have a chance to wreak havoc on our cells. This is one way that minerals help protect us from heart disease, cancer, and other age-related diseases.

Minerals Intake Affects Disease Risk

Mineral intake affects the risk and course of many diseases. For example, researchers have determined that copper deficiency may contribute to high blood pressure, enhanced inflammation, anemia, and heart disease. Low magnesium levels are also associated with heart disease and irregular heartbeats called arrhythmias. Some researchers have compared deficiencies of zinc and some vitamins to harmful radiation because these deficiencies break DNA strands and cause oxidative damage that encourages disease.

As you might expect, sufficient mineral intake can often decrease disease risk and complications. Many studies have found that supplemental calcium decreases a person's risk of osteoporosis, a bone disease affecting millions of people in the United States that causes pain, fracture, and deformity.

Osteoporosis
A disease in which bone loss results in porous bones that are prone to pain, fracture, or deformity.

Zinc has inhibited prostate cancer cell growth and disease progression in recent studies. And it's very clear, based on research results from human clinical trials and other studies, that selenium protects against cancer. Chromium picolinate, the most effective form of the mineral chromium, improves insulin activity and blood glucose levels in people with type 2 diabetes, a disease characterized by high blood sugar levels and an increased risk of heart disease, kidney disease, and nerve function loss.

Supplements Can Boost Mineral Intake

You might be surprised to learn that mineral intake in the United States is often inadequate. Some of the reasons for this are the same as those that explain why people aren't getting enough vitamins: the lack of a truly balanced diet high in vitamins and minerals and lower nutrient levels in farmland soil, for starters.

The good news is that mineral supplements can

help you get enough of these very valuable micronutrients. Certainly, supplements are no substitute for a healthy diet and lifestyle, but they can help fill in nutritional gaps and improve your health. Think of vitamin and mineral supplements as inexpensive insurance.

In the following chapters, you'll read about the important functions of many essential minerals, the latest exciting research about their disease-fighting powers, ways to improve your intake, and where you can learn more about them. The topic of minerals is complex, but if you keep reading, you'll no doubt learn more about how minerals can help you live a long and healthy life.

CHAPTER 8

CALCIUM, MAGNESIUM, AND POTASSIUM FOR HEALTHY HEART AND BONES

You probably already associate calcium with strong bones, but did you know that magnesium is also needed for bone health due to its role in calcium metabolism? Were you aware that calcium can alleviate premenstrual syndrome, that magnesium is recommended for migraine relief, and that potassium might help lower blood pressure? These three minerals have many functions in the body—some related to their common status as electrolytes. Their potential to fend off health problems is promising.

Calcium for Strong Bones and Teeth

Ninety-nine percent of the calcium you ingest is used to mineralize bones and teeth, making them harder and stronger. But the other 1 percent of calcium plays many other roles in health. It helps clot blood, regulates contraction and relaxation in heart and skeletal muscles, frees up energy from food, helps the body use iron, and more.

We tend to view bones as static, solid structures. However, bone is constantly changing, remodeling itself throughout our lives. Calcium absorbed from the diet and supplements is deposited in bone, and old bone is resorbed (the opposite of absorbed) and excreted. Calcium is drawn from bone to normalize body fluid levels when necessary.

People generally reach skeletal maturity and homeostasis by around thirty years of age. This means that the amount of calcium deposited in bone is equal to the amount resorbed. After that, we begin to lose more bone than we gain. This age-related bone loss is associated with the loss of bone strength and density and increased susceptibility to fracture over time.

Adequate intake of calcium and other bone-building nutrients (vitamin D, vitamin K, and magnesium, for example) from childhood on encourages the formation of new bone, protecting us from the bone disease osteoporosis as we age. Ten million people in the United States have the disease, in which bones become porous, fragile, and susceptible to fracture. Eighteen million more are at risk for the disease due to low bone mass.

Menopausal and postmenopausal women are especially at risk for osteoporosis, as bone loss speeds up when estrogen levels decline in menopause. In fact, one in two women over age sixty-five will have an osteoporotic fracture. Building strong bones early in life with good nutrition and regular exercise is paramount to staving off osteoporosis down the road. Adequate calcium intake, in the presence of vitamin D, has been proven to prevent bone loss and reduce the risk of fractures in peri- and postmenopausal women.

Calcium is also useful in treating osteoporosis. In a recent research review of eleven well-designed studies, calcium was effective in treating the disease among populations with low intake who were given adequate supplementation. This mineral may also offer benefits in relation to disorders including hypertension, colorectal cancer, and obesity, but the scope of calcium's effects and the way it works in these disorders are not well understood.

Calcium Can Alleviate PMS

Premenstrual syndrome, or PMS, is one of the most common disorders in women, afflicting millions of premenopausal age. Fortunately, calcium has proven effective in significantly alleviating PMS. Clinical trials have found that calcium supplementation alleviates most mood and physical symptoms, such as cramps.

A study reported in the *American Journal of Obstetrics and Gynecology* in 1998 found that 1,200 milligrams of elemental calcium daily taken as calcium carbonate was effective in squelching PMS symptoms. Several hundred healthy, premenopausal female subjects took the calcium supplements or placebo for the duration of three menstrual cycles. Those taking calcium experienced reduced total symptoms of PMS by 48 percent overall by the third cycle (the placebo group improved only 30 percent). Symptoms reduced included "negative effect," water retention, food cravings, and pain. Although 1,200–1,600 mg per day of calcium supplementation may alleviate PMS, women can take less if they eat diets high in calcium.

It isn't surprising that calcium and PMS are interrelated. Ovarian hormones affect the metabolism of calcium, vitamin D, and magnesium, and calcium metabolism and its intestinal absorption are regulated by estrogen. Fluctuating hormone levels throughout the menstrual cycle affect the regulation of calcium and these other nutrients. PMS shares several symptoms (anxiety and depression, for example) with hypocalcemia, a state of below-normal calcium levels. This has led some researchers to conclude that PMS represents the manifestation of calcium deficiency that can be reversed with supplementation.

Getting Enough Calcium

Most people associate calcium with dairy products, but it is also found in seafood, almonds, sesame seeds, mustard greens, corn tortillas, broccoli, dried fruits, beans, and other foods. Even so, you may not be getting enough calcium. It's one of the few nutrients still deficient in several industrialized countries, including the United States.

The average adult gets 500–700 mg of the recommended 1,000 mg per day for adults over age eighteen. A supplement of 300–700 mg per day may even be sufficient for optimal intake. A dosage of

1,200 mg per day is recommended for women over age fifty on estrogen replacement therapy (ERT), and 1,500 mg is recommended for women not taking ERT. In addition, 400–600 mg of vitamin D is recommended to ensure adequate calcium absorption.

Adolescents aged nine to eighteen should get 1,300 mg of calcium each day. Pregnant and lactating women should follow guidelines for their age group, according to Tori Hudson, N.D., a professor of gynecology at the National College of Naturopathic Medicine in Portland, Oregon. Calcium absorption increases during pregnancy, so higher intake for pregnant women may not be necessary. Up to 2,500 mg of calcium daily is considered safe.

Only about one-third of the calcium you ingest is actually absorbed, and absorption varies among different forms. Dollar for dollar, calcium citrate is the

Chelated Minerals
Minerals that are bound to other molecules that increase absorption by the body.

best-absorbed form. Avoid calcium from oyster shell or bone meal, as these can contain high levels of lead. The lowest lead levels are in refined calcium carbonate and calcium chelates. Citrate, fumarate, malate, succinate, and aspartate are all chelate forms of calcium. Hudson advises taking half the recommended dosage if you're taking calcium citrate or malate, the most absorbable forms.

Antacids are not a good source of calcium for two reasons. One, the aluminum compound they contain may hinder calcium absorption, and two, they may reduce calcium absorption by making the stomach more alkaline. There is also concern that aluminum may be linked to the development of Alzheimer's disease. Research suggests that calcium-rich bottled mineral waters, however, are a good source and at least as well absorbed as that from dairy products.

Too much calcium can interfere with absorption of zinc and other nutrients. For example, magnesium and calcium compete for absorption when there is an excess of either in the gut. Finding a well-formulated multivitamin and mineral supplement or bone health formula can help you get enough—but not too much—of each ingredient. Many experts recommend taking two parts calcium to one part magnesium. Calcium and phosphorous in a ratio of 2:1 in a formula is also often advised.

Magnesium—The Multifaceted Mineral

Magnesium is needed for proper calcium metabolism and deficiencies of it have been linked to osteoporosis. This trace mineral is involved in several hundred chemical reactions in the body and is required by every cell. Magnesium is needed to generate and use adenosine triphosphate, or ATP, your body's energy source. It is also involved in contracting heart and smooth muscle, mineral absorption, protein synthesis, blood clotting, and insulin function.

Sixty percent or more of magnesium in your body is found in bone, so it's not surprising that depleted magnesium levels negatively affect bone metabolism and are considered a risk factor in osteoporosis. Oral magnesium supplements suppressed bone turnover in healthy, young men in one recent study. Because increased bone turnover contributes to bone loss, magnesium supplementation may reduce bone loss associated with high bone turnover, such as in age-related osteoporosis.

Magnesium benefits more than bones. Deficiency of this mineral has been linked to insulin resistance, and supplementation has improved insulin sensitivity and insulin secretion among patients with type 2 diabetes. Insulin helps glucose (the sugar your cells use for fuel) go from blood into cells to be used for energy. This keeps the amount of glucose in blood within a normal range.

In diabetes, the body doesn't produce enough insulin, or cells aren't sensitive to the insulin it does produce. The result is dangerously elevated blood glucose levels. Theoretically, better insulin sensitivity and secretion resulting from magnesium supplementation could help regulate the amount of glucose in blood.

No beneficial effect of magnesium on blood glucose control in diabetic patients has yet been demonstrated, though. Still, there is also potential for magnesium to help people with diabetes by decreasing the risk of retinopathy (deterioration in the blood vessels of the retina) and high blood pressure (at least a little).

Diabetes Mellitus
A condition caused by undersecretion of the hormone insulin (in type 1 diabetes) or cell insensitivity to insulin (in type 2 diabetes), leading to high blood glucose levels.

Many studies have shown that magnesium intake affects blood pressure. High blood pressure is a major risk factor for stroke, the third leading cause of death in the world. Magnesium, as well as potassium and fiber, appeared to decrease stroke risk in male subjects in one study, especially among those who were hypertensive (that is, those who had high blood pressure).

Another study found that diets high in magnesium and potassium were associated with reduced medication cost and better blood pressure control in elderly, hypertensive patients. These findings led researchers to recommend increased magnesium intake for hypertensive people. (Anyone with kidney problems should consult their doctor first.) Magnesium, along with calcium and potassium, encourages relaxation of vascular smooth muscle, helping to keep blood passageways open and blood pressure in check.

Ameliorating Migraines and More

Migraine is marked by extremely painful headaches, nausea, vomiting, increased sensitivity to light and sound, and reduced activity. Drugs used to treat migraine have side effects. Low brain levels of magnesium have been reported in migraine, and as many as 50 percent of patients have lowered levels of ionized magnesium during an attack.

In one recent study, two weeks of magnesium-rich mineral water intake improved intracellular (that is, within cells) magnesium status in migraine patients. Intravenous magnesium sulfate alleviates pain and other symptoms during migraine attacks, but a doctor must administer this form. Two well-controlled studies have suggested that regular oral magnesium supplementation might reduce the frequency of migraine headaches. These supplements are safe, inexpensive, and often recommended for migraine.

Magnesium may also benefit heart failure and heart attack patients, pregnant women with preeclampsia (also called toxemia), chronic fatigue patients, and others under a doctor's guidance. These topics are beyond the scope of this book, but the list does highlight the breadth of magnesium's impact.

Taking More Magnesium

It's difficult to measure a person's magnesium levels, because 99 percent of this mineral in your body is in soft tissue and bone as opposed to blood, which is easier to test. Even so, we know that deficiency is common in the general population. Low levels can result from low intake, diarrhea, vomiting, chronic diuretic use, some prescription medications, and too much sugar and fat in the diet.

Some good dietary sources of magnesium are nuts, legumes, soybeans, blackstrap molasses, vegetables, seafood, and brown rice. When it comes to supplements, look for magnesium in citrate, aspartate, or malate forms. These are better absorbed and tend to not have the laxative effect of magnesium sulfate and others.

The RDA for magnesium is 310–320 mg daily for adult females and 400–420 mg daily for adult men. Up to 700 mg a day may be recommended for specific health problems. Excess magnesium is unlikely to cause toxicity in healthy people. If you have diarrhea from magnesium supplementation, reduce the dosage. Those with kidney disorders should consult their doctors before taking magnesium, as should pregnant and nursing women.

Potassium—Keeping the Body in Balance

Potassium, sodium, calcium, magnesium, and chloride all act as electrolytes in body fluids. The molecules of electrolytes separate into charged ions when dissolved in water, and all electrolytes have either a negative charge (anions) or a positive charge (cations). They control water movement between body compartments, help maintain acid-base balance, and carry electrical current in the body. Potassium is the main cation (remember, a particle with a positive charge) in the fluid inside cells. We all need normal levels for the life of our cells.

Electrolytes *Substances that separate into charged ions when dissolved in water.*

With sodium (another cation), potassium helps keep the body's acid-base balance, or pH in check. The pH is a measure of hydrogen ion concentration in body fluids. Don't worry about the chemistry, just keep in mind that pH must be kept within a limited range to maintain the body's delicate balance, or homeostasis. Potassium also has a diuretic effect, meaning that it encourages your body to excrete water through urination. With sodium (which has the opposite effect), potassium helps balance body fluid levels.

In addition to its role in bone health, energy use, nerve function, normal heartbeat, and more, potassium is known for its ability to lower blood pressure, at least marginally. As noted earlier, dietary intake of potassium and magnesium are associated with keeping blood pressure in check among the elderly. A study published in the *American Journal of Hypertension* found that non-medicated, hypertensive subjects who increased dietary intake of potassium, magnesium, and calcium over ten weeks successfully decreased blood pressure.

Another recent study found that middle-aged male and female Chinese subjects—who tend to eat a diet high in salt and low in potassium—experienced significant reductions in blood pressure with moderate potassium supplementation for ten weeks. Additional study results, published in the journal *Circulation*, showed that potassium supplement use was inversely related to stroke risk among middle-aged men. Supplementation was especially protective in hypertensive men. Longer-term studies are needed to measure the benefit.

Potassium deficiencies are rare, but if you're taking diuretics, laxatives, or corticosteroid drugs or if you have diabetes, you may have depleted levels. Severe vomiting and diarrhea could lead to deficiencies, too. Striving for a ratio of five times as much potassium as sodium in your diet is advised by some experts. There is no RDA for this nutrient, but up to 4,500 mg per day has been recommended to offset high salt intake. You might want to cut back on salt intake, too.

CHAPTER 9

REDUCE YOUR CANCER RISK WITH SELENIUM

Selenium was once regarded as toxic, but now it's considered as an essential dietary mineral. Selenium is a powerful antioxidant that protects against serious health problems, including cancer. It improves vitamin E activity in the body and helps the body hang on to this vital vitamin. Selenium shows promise in limiting heart disease risk (by protecting cholesterol from lipid peroxidation) and more.

Prostate Cancer Prevention

Prostate cancer protection is one of selenium's most well researched benefits. This disease is the second leading cause of cancer deaths in men, so finding a way to fend off this killer is a high public health priority. Selenium falls under the heading of chemopreventive agents, because it seems to ward off cancer before it strikes.

In a 1998 study published in the *British Journal of Urology*, 974 patients with a history of prostate cancer received either 200 micrograms of selenium or a placebo for four and a half years. After six and a half years from the beginning of the study, only thirteen prostate cancer cases in the selenium-treated group had developed, compared to thirty-five cases in the placebo group. The incidence of lung and colorectal cancer was also lower among the

Prostate Gland
The doughnut-shaped gland below the bladder in men that surrounds the upper part of the urethra and secretes a solution that aids in sperm movement and health.

selenium-treated group. Another group of researchers determined that higher, long-term selenium intake was associated with reduced prostate cancer development in several thousand men aged forty to seventy.

Researchers have questioned whether the link between low selenium levels and prostate cancer may simply be due to cancer depleting selenium in the body. In other words, do low selenium levels encourage cancer, or vice versa? But results from many studies measuring long-term supplementation before the onset of cancer suggest that preexisting low selenium levels increased the risk of developing cancer.

More Cancer Protection

The Journal of the National Cancer Institute has reported that pretrial blood selenium levels were inversely associated with the later incidence of esophageal and gastric cardia cancer. Very low selenium status might also contribute to lung cancer risk, according to additional findings. High blood levels of selenium have even been associated with reductions in liver cancer risk among men with chronic hepatitis virus infection.

In a study published in the *European Journal of Clinical Nutrition* in 2001, sixty patients with gastric cancer undergoing chemotherapy were given 200 mcg of selenium daily and 21 mg of zinc daily as tablets for fifty days. The patients taking zinc and selenium had improved conditions (stable nutritional status and increased appetite, for example) by the study's end.

Selenium seems to fight cancer—both before it develops and after it has struck—in more ways than one. Selenomethionine, a common form of this mineral, induced apoptosis, or cell death, in human prostate cancer cells during in vitro studies. Normal human prostate cells were unharmed by selenium.

Other evidence suggests that selenium protects

DNA, fats, and protein in the body from oxidative damage, due to its antioxidant action. Oxidative damage sets the stage for carcinogenesis, or cancer development. Many experts agree that selenium and other antioxidants (including vitamin E) may be beneficial in preventing prostate and other cancers.

Selenium Blocks Dangerous Viruses

Outbreaks of influenza, or flu, kill more than 20,000 Americans each year and hospitalize another 110,000 annually. New strains appear every year, so it's virtually impossible for the immune system to make a permanent defense against flu-causing viruses. But recent research suggests that adequate intake of selenium might prevent dangerous flu virus mutations.

A study conducted by Melinda A. Beck, Ph.D., and her colleagues found that mice eating a low-selenium diet that were exposed to a mild flu virus developed more serious infections than those eating diets with adequate selenium. This flu virus also mutated into another form, making lung infections worse in the selenium-deficient mice and causing infections in healthy mice. Beck and her colleagues had found, in earlier published studies, that mutations in the Coxsackie's virus in Chinese citizens were stimulated by deficiencies in selenium.

Selenium and zinc supplementation boosted immune function in a two-year study of 725 French geriatric patients, published in *The Archives of Internal Medicine* in 1999. Subjects receiving low-dose zinc and selenium developed increased levels of infection-fighting antibodies and fewer respiratory tract infections. Subjects taking low-dose vitamin supplements instead didn't experience these benefits.

The effects of selenium on immunity help explain why the mineral may protect us from flu and cancer. Selenium is needed for the production of glutathione peroxidase, a powerful antioxidant and immune-system stimulant. Inadequate levels of selenium disable the body's antioxidant defenses. This breakdown seems to allow free radicals to mutate otherwise-stable DNA.

Selenium deficiencies might also decrease the body's production of natural killer cells. These are a kind of lymphocyte, or immune cell, that targets and destroys tumor- or virus-infected cells. Selenium and zinc deficiencies among elderly people have been linked to low natural killer cell levels. This immune activity might explain why HIV and AIDS patients are thought to benefit from selenium supplementation.

> **Natural-Killer Cells**
> *A type of immune cell that targets and destroys tumor- or virus-infected cells.*

Supplementing with Selenium

Bran, garlic (from selenium-rich soil), oatmeal, onions, mushrooms, broccoli, brown rice, and whole-grain products are plant sources of selenium. Eggs, tuna, seafood, chicken, and liver are good animal sources of the mineral. Even so, low soil levels of selenium and food processing can lead to inadequate amounts in the diet.

Supplements can help you get enough selenium. Both selenomethionine and high-selenium yeast are excellent supplements, and the high-selenium yeast has been found to reduce the risk of several types of cancer in people. A daily dosage of 200 mcg is considered safe and adequate for the average American adult.

Very high doses of selenium—more than 800 mcg daily or more for extended periods—could be hazardous. Follow recommended intakes to reap only the benefits of selenium. Deficiencies are more likely, and they can lead to nerve disorders, early aging, increased fragility of red blood cells, pancreatic degeneration, and weakened vision.

CHAPTER 10

CHROMIUM OPTIMIZES INSULIN AND GLUCOSE FUNCTION

Chromium is a trace mineral that you need for normal sugar and fat metabolism. It improves the efficiency of insulin, a hormone that orchestrates the movement of sugar and fat into your body's cells to be used or stored for energy. When chromium levels are low, insulin can't perform well. This can set the stage for diabetes mellitus, obesity, and heart disease. Increasing daily intake of this essential element can help control diabetes and may aid in weight loss and lowering cholesterol levels.

Improving Insulin Efficiency

Several clinical studies have shown that chromium supplements improve insulin activity in people with diabetes. This is good news, because low insulin production and insulin insensitivity are serious problems in the all too common disorder. The most promising results have been in regard to type 2 (or non-insulin dependent) diabetes. Unlike people with the type 1 (insulin-dependent) diabetes, those with type 2 diabetes produce enough insulin in their bodies. The problem is that their cells' insulin receptors aren't sensitive to insulin.

Insulin
A hormone that helps move sugar and fat from blood into body cells to be used or stored for energy.

When the body doesn't produce enough insulin (as in type 1) or cell receptors aren't sensitive to the hormone (as in type 2), glucose can't be ushered into cells from the bloodstream. Instead, blood glucose levels remain dangerously high and cells don't receive the fuel they need. This leads to serious health problems.

Numerous studies have found that supplemental chromium, in the form of chromium picolinate, improves blood glucose, insulin, and cholesterol status among people with type 2 diabetes, who tend to have low chromium levels. No side effects have been documented among people with type 2 diabetes taking supplemental chromium.

A lack of chromium seems to increase the risk of insulin resistance, a condition also called Syndrome X. In Syndrome X the body can't process glucose normally, so it secretes more and more insulin. The insulin does not work efficiently, so it keeps circulating in the blood along with the elevated blood levels of glucose. Syndrome X, which is characterized by insulin resistance and abdominal obesity, greatly increases risk of heart disease and diabetes. Some experts estimate that 25 percent of the population suffers from Syndrome X, with most cases undiagnosed.

Syndrome X
A disorder marked by high blood levels of insulin and glucose and associated with high cholesterol and other blood fat levels and with increased risk of heart disease and diabetes.

Insulin becomes less effective when we eat a lot of sugary foods and refined carbohydrates, such as sweets, pasta, and white bread. When we eat too much of these foods, muscle cells temporarily switch off their insulin recognition system. As a result, blood sugar, or blood glucose, is redirected to fat cells and to the liver. Eventually, fat cells ignore insulin altogether; they become insulin-resistant.

When cells stop pulling glucose out of the blood, the glucose spills over into the urine. This is a typical sign of diabetes. However, a person can have trouble with insulin and insulin resistance, or Syndrome X, without being diabetic. Chromium deficiency is characterized by many of the signs of Syndrome X, including insulin resistance, poor glucose control, and high cholesterol and triglyceride levels.

Several studies have found that chromium picolinate supplementation can play a major role in reducing symptoms of Syndrome X and diabetes. Again, chromium works by enhancing insulin function and the burning of blood sugar, or glucose. Chromium supplements alone are not a cure for Syndrome X, but they can help reverse this disorder.

Chromium and Lean Body Mass

Chromium is purported to spare or increase lean body mass and aid in fat loss. Some—but not all—research does support the theory that chromium may help those looking to increase (or keep) muscle and lose fat. Considering chromium's role in sugar and fat metabolism, it does seem plausible.

In a recent double-blind, placebo-controlled study, twenty overweight African-American women followed a modest diet and exercise regimen and received either placebo or 200 mcg of chromium (in the niacin-bound form) three times daily for two months. Then, they switched to the other regime for two months. Body weight loss was comparable with both regimens, but fat loss was greater and lean body mass loss was less with chromium intake compared to placebo. The women had lost more fat and less muscle by taking 600 mcg of niacin-bound chromium daily, experiencing no adverse effects.

In another double-blind study, 123 participants took either a patented natural dietary supplement containing chromium picolinate, inulin (a long-chain sugar molecule found in Jerusalem artichokes), capsicum, L-phenylalanine (a protein building block), and other potentially fat-fighting nutrients or placebo for four weeks. They all followed the same diet and exercise program throughout the study. At the end of the study, those taking the natural supplement had a faster rate of body fat loss and maintained more lean body mass than the placebo group.

Of course, this study didn't investigate the effects of chromium alone. And eating a healthy diet and exercising are crucial to any fat- and weight-loss plan, as they were in these studies. Even so, there appears to be potential for chromium to play a role in decreasing one's fat to muscle ratio. Future large-scale human trials should shed more light on the topic, as well as on the potential for chromium supplementation to decrease total and LDL, or "bad," cholesterol levels.

Choosing Supplements

Normal dietary intake of chromium is often less than optimal. Mushrooms, prunes, nuts, asparagus, organ meats, and whole-grain products are good sources, but levels of chromium in these foods vary. Chromium supplements have an excellent safety record and are relatively inexpensive.

The amount of chromium a person needs depends on age, activity level, and overall health. For example, a teenaged girl might benefit from 200–300 mcg daily, whereas 300–400 mcg daily may be best for a teenaged boy. Adults up to retirement age should get 400 mcg daily. Elderly people should take at least 200 mcg per day. The most dramatic and consistent results have been with 200 mcg of chromium picolinate for every 1,000 calories of food eaten.

Some studies have found that 1,000 mcg of chromium daily as chromium picolinate can help patients with diabetes. A daily intake of 200 mcg per day is thought to be enough to improve glucose tolerance in people who do not have full-blown diabetes. Anyone with diabetes should work with a doctor on this, however, because insulin or hypoglycemic drug requirements may need to be adjusted.

Chromium picolinate is made up of chromium combined chemically with picolinic acid in order to help the body use it most efficiently, so choose a supplement with this form. Chromium picolinate is sometimes referred to as "trivalent" because it is a chelate made of chromium attached to three picolinate molecules.

CHAPTER 11

ZINC AND COPPER FOR IMMUNITY

Zinc is essential to many enzyme systems in the body. We need it to grow and develop, digest protein, produce energy, and absorb vitamin A efficiently, for starters. Prostate and reproductive health depend on adequate zinc status, too. But this mineral is perhaps most famous for its starring role in immune system function. High levels of copper, also an essential mineral, can suppress zinc levels.

Zinc for Immunity

The immune system needs zinc to fight infections. It is required for normal synthesis of deoxyribonucleic acid (DNA), which helps make new immune cells. It also promotes the activity of immune cells. Zinc deficiency leads to impaired immunity and, as a result, increased susceptibility to viral, bacterial, and fungal infections. Infections can even lead to death when the immune system is damaged.

Supplementation with zinc has repeatedly improved immunity in people with low levels. Studies have found that elderly people, who often have low zinc levels, experience a decreased risk of infection by taking the RDA of zinc for one to two months. Zinc and selenium supplements have improved immunity and decreased the risk of respiratory infections among elderly patients. Zinc also increases the survival rate of elderly people following infection.

Children need zinc for strong immunity, too. In a recent study, Indian researchers gave 609 children, ranging in age from six months to three years, daily supplements of zinc gluconate (containing 10 mg of elemental zinc) or a multivitamin without zinc. After four months of supplementation, zinc levels increased in children receiving zinc. Levels declined in the other group. Children taking zinc had a 45 percent reduction in acute lower respiratory infections.

Results with zinc lozenges for cold symptom relief have been mixed, but many have concluded that these lozenges in the gluconate or acetate forms reduce the symptoms and duration of colds. In one recent study, fifty patients who began taking zinc acetate lozenges (containing 12.8 mg of zinc) every two to three hours within twenty-four hours of the onset of cold symptoms reported symptom relief in less than five days, compared to eight days for symptom relief among the placebo group.

Zinc's role in immunity helps explain its ability to inactivate viruses (including some types of herpes). The immune-boosting mineral is sometimes recommended to patients with the AIDS virus (along with conventional drug therapy), who often have low levels and hindered immune function. It works by inactivating a protease that is essential for the proliferation of the AIDS virus HIV-1. Zinc may also offer protection against various forms of cancer, due in part to its positive effects on the immune system.

Prostate Cancer Protection and Then Some

Healthy prostate tissue has the highest zinc levels of any body soft tissue. This suggests that it plays a big role in the prostate. Cancer protection may be part of that role.

Zinc levels in prostate cancer are significantly decreased compared to levels in other tissues. A recent human cell culture study published in the journal *Prostate* revealed that zinc prompted self-destruction (apoptosis) and inhibited growth of human prostate cancer cells. Another study—this one with 697 men with prostate cancer—found that the subjects had low supplement intake of zinc and vitamins C and E individually over the two years before their cancer diagnosis. Researchers concluded that each of these three supplements might have a protective effect against prostate cancer. There is strong evidence that the loss of the ability to hang on to zinc is a factor in the development and progression of prostate cancer cells.

Zinc is needed for sexual maturation and reproduction, including the production of the hormone testosterone and sperm formation. Infertile males tend to have lower levels of zinc than fertile males, and low blood levels of testosterone have been linked to low zinc levels. What's more, this antioxidant mineral may work by scavenging free radicals produced by defective sperm in semen after ejaculation, according to study results. It is crucial in maintaining prostate and testicular tissue.

Heart health is another promising area of zinc research. Zinc protects cell walls, and it appears to protect blood vessel walls from injury that can contribute to atherosclerosis, or hardening of the arteries. In addition, a dose of 25 mg of zinc daily for three months decreased oxidation of blood fats during a recent study of elderly Italian men and women. (Remember that oxidized blood fats can eventually lead to blockage of blood flow.) The researchers concluded that adequate intake could be important in preventing and regulating age-related diseases.

Atherosclerosis
Describes the buildup of blood fats on the damaged lining of artery walls, leading to plaques that block blood flow.

Another study found that zinc intake was positively associated with a healthier ratio of total cholesterol to HDL, or "good" cholesterol, among African-American male subjects. (A high ratio of HDL to total cholesterol is desirable.) Female African-American subjects with higher zinc intake had higher HDL values than subjects with low intake. In other words, zinc might protect against heart disease by improving cholesterol levels. Study results with European Americans have been mixed.

The effect of zinc supplementation in Wilson's disease is clearer. The FDA even approved zinc acetate for treatment of the disease, which results in the toxic buildup of copper in the body, liver disease, and neurological disorders. The two FDA-approved treatment drugs for Wilson's disease have side effects and may damage fetuses. In a recent study, zinc was found to be effective and safe for mothers and fetuses. (Consult your doctor first if you're pregnant or nursing.) It works by inducing intestinal metallothionein, which binds to copper and keeps it from entering the blood.

Ensuring Adequate Intake

There are some good sources of zinc in the food we eat—pumpkin seeds, turkey, whole grains, and raw oysters, for example. But you may need more. Researchers from the Centers for Disease Control and Prevention found that only slightly more than half of Americans surveyed in the Third National Health and Nutrition Examination Survey got adequate amounts of zinc from food and supplements. Children aged one to three years old, adolescent girls, and people over age seventy-one were at greatest risk of inadequate intake.

Some signs of zinc deficiency are growth retardation, loss of appetite, diarrhea, impotence, and increased risk of infectious diseases. The RDA is 8 mg per day for women and 11 mg per day for men, but some practitioners recommend up to 50 mg per day. Taking much more than that regularly can cause signs of toxicity, including diarrhea and upset stomach.

Look for citrate, gluconate, or protein chelate forms of zinc. When it comes to lozenges, opt for those supplying 15–25 mg of elemental zinc per lozenge. Choose a brand sweetened with glycine, as other sweeteners (sorbitol, mannitol, and citric acid) might limit absorption. Dissolve them in your mouth every couple of hours for up to seven days when you feel a cold coming on.

Be Sure to Get Some Copper

Copper activates key enzyme reactions and helps make ATP, the body's energy source. It is, along with zinc, part of an antioxidant enzyme called superoxide dismutase, or SOD, which keeps free radical damage in check. Copper is involved in making hormones and collagen, a protein that holds connective tissue together. It is also needed to make hemoglobin, the molecule that carries oxygen in the blood.

A potential benefit of copper supplementation is its ability to relieve inflammation and ease symptoms of rheumatoid arthritis. Animal studies have found that a copper-supplemented diet has an antiarthritic effect, but human studies are lacking. Increased body copper levels, which are associated with arthritis inflammation, were once thought to make the disease worse. But now they are thought to increase as part of the body's response to arthritis.

Getting enough copper may help your heart, too. Copper deficiency might hamper heart health by contributing to high blood pressure, increased inflammation, arteriosclerosis, and anemia. Inadequate copper reduces the effectiveness of many enzymes, so deficiencies can lead to negative changes in the heart, blood vessels, and circulating blood cells, according to authors of a research review published in the journal *Biofactors*.

Most people get enough copper because it is in so many foods. Multivitamin and mineral supplements also contain it. You should only take extra copper if your doctor recommends it, as toxicity can occur at high levels. People taking large amounts of zinc may need 1–2 mg of copper per day.

CHAPTER 12

IRON, IODINE, AND MANGANESE

Several minor minerals play essential roles in health. Of these, iron and iodine are well known to most people, but manganese is not. This chapter describes some of their important roles in maintaining health.

Iron for Life—In Small Amounts

The micromineral iron is part of hemoglobin, the protein that transports oxygen in red blood cells to other body cells that need it. Iron is also part of myoglobin, which supplies oxygen to muscles. It is needed to make ATP, as well. People deficient in this mineral tire easily because their bodies' cells aren't getting the oxygen they need, or they aren't synthesizing enough ATP for energy.

Most of us grew up hearing about how important it is to get enough iron. Iron is essential to life itself, but it may surprise you to learn that most adults don't need supplemental iron. In fact, too much iron can cause oxidative damage.

This kind of damage can contribute to or worsen some diseases (including heart disease, and rheumatoid arthritis) and speed up aging, so it's best not to supplement with iron unless you know that you're deficient. Some research results even suggest that iron overload, or hemochromatosis, may contribute to the risk of developing heart disease in men and women, due to the mineral's role in increasing oxidation.

Monthly blood losses of iron in premenopausal

women actually protect against iron overload. After menopause, women no longer lose iron on a monthly basis, so they can end up with high levels. This relationship may help explain why postmenopausal women have a higher risk of heart disease than their younger counterparts.

Deficiency and Dosage

People who are deficient in iron usually lose large amounts or don't absorb iron well, as opposed to merely having a low intake. Pregnant and lactating women, infants and children, elderly people, endurance athletes, and people with hemorrhoids, ulcerative colitis, or other conditions might be at risk. Even these people should check with their doctors before starting an iron supplement routine beyond a multivitamin and mineral formula.

Women who have very heavy menstrual periods might have low iron levels, too. That's because iron is lost in menstrual blood every month. But the amount found in a multivitamin and mineral formula helps restore lost iron in these women.

Anemia
A blood condition in which the amount of hemoglobin in red blood cells, or the number of red blood cells themselves, is below normal.

Iron-deficiency anemia does sometimes result from iron deficiency. In this disorder, hemoglobin in blood cells, or the number of red blood cells themselves, is low. If you experience fatigue and have trouble breathing normally, consult your doctor to determine whether or not you have anemia and if it is caused by iron deficiency or another problem. Do not try to self-treat what you think may be anemia.

The most absorbable iron, called heme iron, is found in clams, oysters, red meat, and organ meats. Dark, leafy green vegetables, brewer's yeast, wheat germ, blackstrap molasses, and acidic foods cooked in iron pans are sources of non-heme iron. Vegetarians may have lower iron levels than meat-eaters because iron from plant sources is less absorbable; however, many non-meat foods, such as cereal, are fortified with iron. Vitamin C can aid iron absorption, too, so drinking orange juice with your cereal, for example, increases absorption.

If you're concerned about heart disease risk, consider taking an iron-free multivitamin and supplement formula. For premenopausal women, an iron-containing multivitamin and mineral formula is probably a good idea. Iron toxicity is very dangerous and especially serious in children, so stick to the RDA.

Iodine for Thyroid Health

Iodine and the amino acid tyrosine are required by the thyroid gland in order to secrete thyroid hormones, which regulate biochemical reactions. In the early 1900s, low iodine levels in soil and water led to hypothyroidism and goiter (enlarged thyroid) among people living in Michigan and other "goiter belt" states. Thanks to the addition of iodine to table salt, deficiencies are rare in the United States today.

Iodine deficiency and hypothyroidism are much more common in developing countries, where people don't consume iodized salt. A deficiency can result in mental retardation, goiter, abnormal development, and cretinism, a serious developmental disorder in infants. Some studies and clinical findings suggest a link between low iodine intake and fibrocystic breasts, a condition causing breast pain, discomfort, and/or lumpiness. Increased iodine intake and other natural remedies may improve fibrocystic breasts. Talk to a nutritionally minded doctor if this affects you.

The RDA for iodine is 150 mcg for adults, but the average intake in the United States is more than 600 mcg per day. It's best not to get more than 600 mcg per day on a regular basis, as high levels may hinder normal thyroid function.

Manganese Aids Cartilage Formation

Manganese is necessary for normal brain function, collagen formation, bone growth, energy metabolism, and more. It is only found in trace amounts in people—about 10–20 mg total in the average man. It is not related to magnesium.

There's a chance that this trace mineral may improve arthritis and diabetes in people with low levels, but more human studies are needed. Animal studies have found that manganese is involved in making chondroitin sulfate, a part of articular cartilage and a common supplement for arthritis relief. Deficiencies of manganese have caused a disorder of cartilage metabolism in farm animals. Whether or not low manganese intake contributes to arthritis, and whether supplementation can alleviate arthritis in people, remains to be seen.

Manganese is part of the antioxidant enzyme MnSOD. (This is another form of SOD, which we mentioned earlier.) This enzyme is part of the body's defense against harmful free radical damage to pancreas beta cells, which normally produce insulin but don't work well in type 1 diabetes. Manganese is needed by SOD to protect against free radical damage to insulin-producing cells. (Low levels of MnSOD have been found in patients with osteoarthritis, too.)

In guinea pigs, manganese deficiency leads to diabetes and pancreas abnormalities in their offspring. Low levels of manganese are common in people with diabetes. Even so, future human studies are needed to find out whether or not manganese is effective as diabetes therapy.

Deficiencies of manganese are very rare and there is no RDA. A daily intake of 1.8 mg for women and 2.3 mg for men is considered adequate. Whole grains, fruits, nuts, and vegetables are high in manganese.

CHAPTER 13

SULFUR, SILICON, AND VANADIUM

Relatively little is known about the minerals sulfur, silicon, and vanadium, but they do play crucial roles in health. For example, sulfur is one of the most abundant minerals in the body, but most nutrition textbooks do not discuss it at all. Without sulfur, life simply would not be possible. Why it has been so ignored is a mystery.

Sulfur for Skin and Maybe More

Sulfur is a component of amino acids and thiamine, biotin, lipoic acid, and some hormones, including insulin. It has been used therapeutically for thousands of years to treat skin disorders, such as eczema and psoriasis. Sulfur baths are still recommended to people with these conditions.

Like benzoyl peroxide, sulfur is an antiseptic, but it is gentler on the skin. The FDA has even approved sulfur for treating acne. Sulfur is also very safe. Look for topical products containing at least 3 percent sulfur for the best results. (Vitamin E, vitamin A, and other nutrients might alleviate acne, too.)

Low levels of sulfur have been found in arthritis sufferers. Some researchers speculate that increasing sulfur-rich foods in the diet might lessen the pain and swelling associated with arthritis. One recent study published in the journal *Rheumatology International* in 2000 found that sulfur baths prolonged the benefits of sun exposure and Dead Sea mineral-bath treatment (also available at health and natural food stores) among patients with psoriatic arthritis, a type of arthritis associated with the skin condition psoriasis.

A form of sulfur known as methylsulfonylmethane, or MSM, has become popular in the last few years in supplement form, especially in joint health formulas. Stanley Jacob, M.D., of Oregon Health Sciences University, Portland, has found MSM supplements useful in reducing muscle and joint pain and interstitial cystitis (a type of very painful bladder inflammation). According to Jacob, MSM also eases symptoms of scleroderma, a chronic degenerative disease that scars skin, joints, and connective tissue.

Silicon—Micromineral Newcomer

Silicon is needed for normal growth and development of collagen, the "tissue cement" that literally holds together skin, nails, and all of the other tissues in the body. It also helps form cartilage and bone, the latter by speeding up the mineralization of bone.

Silicon, sometimes referred to as silica (silicon dioxide), is considered a sister element to carbon, which forms the basis of all life on Earth. Despite the relative obscurity of silicon, the body contains a higher level of it than it does iron, zinc, copper, and iodine.

Scientists realized, about a century ago, that high levels of silicon were found in tendons, connective tissue, and the eyes, and that it might protect blood vessels against disease. More recent research, while not conclusive, hints that it might lower blood fats and block aluminum absorption in the brain. Recently, researchers have found that the silica form of the mineral can reduce cracking and brittleness in fingernails and improve the appearance of hair.

Vanadium—Looking Ahead

Vanadium is involved in bone and teeth metabolism. It may be needed for good health by humans (as it is in animals). Good food sources include shellfish, spinach, parsley, whole grains, mushrooms, and soy.

No deficiency in humans is known, and there's no RDA, so you don't have to take extra vanadium. Side effects and negative reactions are not likely to be a problem.

Over the last few years, vanadium has garnered attention for its potential to improve diabetes. Several animal and limited human studies testing this relationship have taken place, with promising results. In one study, a combination of vanadium and insulin regenerated beta cells (which make insulin) and relieved diabetes in insulin-dependent diabetic rats during a year of treatment and after treatment ended. Those rats that were given only insulin did not experience these benefits.

Vanadium has proven therapeutic in clinical studies with patients with type 1 diabetes and in others with type 2 diabetes, noted the authors of a recent review published in *The Journal of Complementary Medicine*. The mineral is considered an "insulin mimic," in that it can partially substitute for insulin and help metabolize blood sugar.

However, this benefit, which improves insulin function and lowers blood sugar levels, warrants caution. High-dose vanadium may be toxic, and it may trigger insulin resistance when supplementation is ceased. If you have diabetes, it would be best to discuss vanadium with your physician before you start supplementing with it.

CHAPTER 14

HOW TO BUY QUALITY SUPPLEMENTS

There's no doubt that vitamin and mineral supplements are good for your health. But how do you know which ones to take, how much to take, and in what form? This chapter will steer you in the right direction.

Micronutrients Work as a Team

Vitamins and minerals are essential nutrients, and each performs myriad functions in the body. For example, vitamin C, vitamin E, and folic acid reduce the risk of coronary heart disease. But they protect the heart and blood vessels in different ways. Similarly, vitamin C and the B vitamins can ease arthritis, but they do so differently.

Various vitamins and minerals need other nutrients to do their jobs well. Vitamin D is essential for efficient calcium absorption. Vitamin C encourages iron absorption.

You can improve your health by taking vitamin C supplements, but you could improve it even more by also taking vitamin E supplements. The most sensible approach is to take all of the vitamins and essential minerals. If it's a hassle to take pills, stick with one high-potency multivitamin and mineral supplement.

Set Clear Goals

Set clear objectives that you want to achieve with supplements. If you are in your twenties, eat a reasonably good diet, and are in good health, your objective might be "dietary insurance." A high-potency multivitamin and mineral supplement may be enough. If you're in your thirties or forties and face a lot of stress at home or at work, "stress management" might be an objective. In this case, you might do well taking a high-potency B-complex supplement.

Reducing disease risk is a very clear objective. If people in your family have a high risk of developing heart disease or cancer, it's wise to start supplementing before the first signs of trouble. In addition to a multivitamin, vitamin E would probably be the most important vitamin for you.

If you have specific health problems, such as high blood pressure, hardening of the arteries, premenstrual syndrome (PMS), or osteoporosis, taking high doses of specific supplements may be in order. (Again, check with your doctor first if you have serious health problems or are taking medication.) By starting with specific objectives, you've got something against which to measure your improvement.

How Much and When?

Understanding supplement labels requires knowing a few measurement terms. Most stand for the weight of a given ingredient. For example, g stands for gram, mg for milligram, and mcg for microgram.

To put these weights into perspective, consider that there are about 454 grams in a pound; 1,000 mg in a gram; and 1,000 mcg in a milligram. So, in general, we're talking about very small quantities. For example, 400 mcg of folic acid is equivalent to about $1/70,000$ of an ounce—a very small quantity, but very important nonetheless. IU stands for international unit, which is a way of measuring vitamins A, D, and E. (Unfortunately, international units do not consistently correspond to milligrams.)

Specific recommendations for supplement dosage vary, but you might strive for something similar to the following in a high-potency multivitamin and mineral supplement. To get these amounts, you may have to take more than one tablet or capsule daily.

Vitamin A: 5,000 IU and/or natural
    beta-carotene: 10 mg or 16,000 IU
Vitamin B_1 (thiamine): 10–15 mg
Vitamin B_2 (riboflavin): 10–25 mg
Vitamin B_3 (niacinamide): 100–200 mg
Vitamin B_6 (pyridoxine): 10–20 mg
Vitamin B_{12}: 10–100 mg
Folic acid: 400 mcg
Pantothenic acid: 25–100 mg
Biotin: 30–50 mcg
PABA: 30–50 mg
Choline: 250 mg
Inositol: 250 mg
Vitamin C: 1,000–4,000 mg
Vitamin D: 400 IU
Vitamin E: 400 IU
Vitamin K: 100 mcg

Calcium (citrate or malate): 1,000 mg
Magnesium: 400 mg
Potassium: 99 mg
Selenium: 200 mcg
Chromium (picolinate): 200–400 mcg
Zinc (citrate or gluconate): 15–25 mg
Copper: 1–2 mg
Iron: 18 mg for menstruating women
    (Men should take an iron-free supplement
    unless tests have indicated anemia.)
Iodine: 150 mcg
Manganese: 2–5 mg

These dosages are for adults. Tailoring vitamin and mineral supplements for children can be trickier because they weigh less. For general supplementation, one or two times the children's RDA (which is lower than the adult RDA) should be safe. Stick with RDA levels of vitamins A and D and minerals for children. An easy solution is one of the many children's supplements available at health food stores.

Most multivitamin and mineral formulas contain all of the vitamins and essential minerals, but there is great variation in dosage. Because the RDA is a conservative amount, look for a supplement that provides at least four times the RDA for the B vitamins, vitamin C, and vitamin E. However, stick with RDA levels for vitamins A and D and iron.

Vitamins and minerals are components of food, so in general they are best taken with food. It's a good idea to take them with breakfast so your body can use them while you're most active. If you take your vitamins before going to bed, you may have a restless night, due to their stimulatory effects. Sometimes, product labels recommend taking supplements two or three times a day, with each meal. Some minerals and mineral formulas advise taking them a couple of hours after meals so they won't hinder digestion. Follow label directions for the best results.

If you're taking large amounts of a single vitamin or mineral, it's best to divide the dose over the course of a day. Splitting up the dose improves the efficiency of absorption, so less is excreted. You don't have to take vitamin C with food because it's water-soluble and easily absorbed. Dividing the dose of vitamin C will also reduce the likelihood of loose bowels resulting from taking too much at one time.

Vitamins & Minerals during Pregnancy

If you're a pregnant woman already taking a high-potency multivitamin and mineral formula roughly equivalent to the one outlined above, you're probably fine, though you should show the bottle to your physician to make sure he or she agrees.

While the vitamin levels above are safe, you and your physician may wish to adjust or reduce some of the vitamin or mineral levels. If you are not already taking supplements, consider starting with a prenatal supplement. Ideally, the time to take such a supplement is before you become pregnant. That's because the risk of birth defects is greatest very early in a pregnancy, often before a woman even realizes she is pregnant.

Vitamins are essential for normal fetus development. For example, if the fetus does not have adequate folic acid through its mother's diet by the sixteenth week of pregnancy, its neural tube (spine) will not seal. The result will be a serious birth defect, such as spina bifida.

Also, a study described in the *Journal of the National Cancer Institute* found that women who took vitamins while pregnant were less likely to have children with brain tumors. Of course, it's also important to seek prenatal medical care, eat a balanced diet, and not smoke or drink alcohol during pregnancy.

Natural versus Synthetic

Most vitamin supplements are synthetic duplicates of their natural counterparts in all respects. But there are big differences between natural and synthetic vitamin E and beta-carotene, with the natural form superior to the synthetic. The natural form of vitamin E (d-alpha tocopherol) is twice as well absorbed as the synthetic form (dl-alpha-tocopherol).

Natural beta-carotene supplements are derived from *Dunaliella salina* algae. (This should be listed on the label.) Natural beta-carotene consists of two forms that chemists call isomers. The synthetic form contains only one of these forms.

Vitamin C is produced from corn sugar (dextrose), and the B vitamins are produced through bacterial fermentation. This means that bacteria are cultivated to produce large amounts of B vitamins. Vitamins A, D, and K come from both natural and synthetic sources, but the differences are not significant.

Are Excipients Safe?

All tablets and capsules contain excipients, which are compounds with no nutritional value. They are added to improve the consistency of vitamin supplements during processing.

Before vitamins are pressed into tablets or poured into capsules, they are in powder form and are thoroughly mixed in vats. Some excipients, such as lubricants, promote consistent mixing, so you get the same amount of a vitamin in every tablet or capsule. Other excipients, such as cellulose, add bulk so vitamins can be pressed into tablets. Cellulose also absorbs water, so the tablet swells and breaks apart in your digestive tract.

All excipients are approved for use by the Food and Drug Administration and are safe. Some people, however, may have reactions to specific excipients, such as lactose (milk sugar). If this happens, buy a different product. If you're allergic to milk or you're lactose intolerant, avoid supplements

> **Excipients**
> *Nonnutritive ingredients added to supplements to improve consistency and other characteristics.*

containing lactose. The same goes for corn, yeast, and other potential allergens. In general, capsules contain fewer excipients compared with tablets, and health food store brands tend to have fewer excipients overall than pharmacy brands.

Finding the Best Form

Every supplement form—capsules, tablets, and liquids—has pros and cons. Choosing one over another depends on a variety of factors. Among these are availability, cost, ease of swallowing, digestive efficiency, and the number of excipients you're willing to ingest.

Most supplements are sold in tablet form. They're less expensive to make than capsules, but capsules are easier to swallow than tablets (especially large tablets). One drawback is that sometimes tablets pass through the gut without breaking down. If this happens to you consistently, switch to a capsule, or consider taking betaine hydrochloride or another digestive aid to improve your stomach acid. Tablets can be a good alternative for vegetarians avoiding gelatin capsules (but there are vegetarian capsules out there, too).

Some supplements, such as vitamin B_{12}, are available as sublingual tablets. These are meant to dissolve under the tongue; much the way nitroglycerin (a heart medication) is taken. A network of blood vessels under the tongue instantly absorbs vitamins and drugs. In addition, you'll also find some vitamins and minerals in liquid form. Because vitamins generally don't taste very good, some products contain a lot of sugar to mask the taste.

Time-release Supplements
A supplement manufactured for the slow release of its ingredient(s).

Time-release supplements are another option. The idea behind them is that they maintain steadier levels in the blood and less is excreted. The disadvantage is the cost of time-release supplements; some are twice the cost of regular vitamin supplements. A less expensive approach would be to divide your vitamins into smaller doses that you take throughout the day.

Gauging Results

If you're taking a specific supplement to treat a condition—such as B vitamins to treat arthritis—you should see some benefits within about thirty days, assuming you're taking enough. If you don't see an improvement after thirty days, stop taking the supplement. It's possible that your improvement was very subtle and you won't notice it until you stop. Or maybe you would benefit from a different vitamin.

It's a little harder to assess the effects of vitamins and minerals if you are in good health and are trying to reduce your long-term risk of disease, such as heart disease. The benefits of vitamin and mineral supplements will become clearer the longer you take them. You'll find that you'll be in generally better health than people your age who don't take them.

Also, keep in mind that supplements are supplements to—not replacements for—good nutrition. They provide dietary insurance, they can compensate somewhat for some subtle biological defects, and they can prevent and treat many diseases. But they won't protect you from a fundamentally bad diet. Eat well, and take your supplements.

SELECTED REFERENCES

Anderson, RA. Chromium, glucose intolerance and diabetes. *J Am Coll Nutr*, 1998; 17(6):548–555.

Badmaev, V, Prakash, S, Majeed, M. Vanadium: a review of its potential role in the fight against diabetes. *J Altern Complement Med*, 1999; 5(3):273–291.

Burton, GW, Traber, MG, Acuff, RV, et al. Human plasma and tissue a-tocopherol concentrations in response to supplementation with deuterated natural and synthetic vitamin E. *American Journal of Clinical Nutrition*, 1998; 67: 669–684.

Bohmer, H, Muller, H, Resch, KL. Calcium supplementation with calcium-rich mineral waters: a systematic review and meta-analysis of its bioavailability. *Osteoporosis Int*, 2000; 11(11):938–943.

Cathcart, RF. Vitamin C, titrating to bowel tolerance, anascorbemia, and acute induced scurvy. *Medical Hypotheses*, 1981; 7:1359–1376.

Clark, LC, Dalkin, B, Krongrad, A, et al. Decreased incidence of prostate cancer with selenium supplementation: results of a double-blind cancer prevention trial. *Br J Urol*, 1998; 81(5):730–734.

Crawford, V, Scheckenbach, R, Preuss, HG. Effects of niacin-bound chromium supplementation on body composition in overweight African-American women. *Diabetes Obes Metab*, 1999; 1(6):331–337.

Douglas, RM, Chalker, EB, Treacy, B. Vitamin C for preventing and treating the common cold. *Cochrane Database Syst Rev*, 2000; 2:CD000980.

Eberlein-Kinig, B, Placzek,M, Pryzybill, B. Protective effect against sunburn of combined systemic ascorbic acid (vitamin C) and d-a-tocopherol (vitamin E). *Journal of the American Academy of Dermatology*, 1998:45–48.

Hoeger, WW, Harris, C, Long, EM, et al. Four-week supplementation with a natural dietary compound produces favorable changes in body composition. *Adv Ther*, 1998; 15(5):305–314.

Jacques, PF, Taylor, A, Hankinson, SF, et al. Long-term vitamin C supplement use and prevalence of early age-related lens opacities. *American Journal of Clinical Nutrition*, 1997; 66:911–916.

Jialal, I, Traber, M, Deveraj, S. Is there a vitamin E paradox? Current Opinion in Lipidology, 2001; 12:49–53.

Keniston, RC, Nathan, PA, Leklem, JE, et al. Vitamin B6, vitamin C, and carpal tunnel syndrome. *Journal of Occupational and Environmental Medicine*, 1997; 949–959.

LéCone, J, Delhinger, V, Maes, D, et al. *Revue Du Rhumatisme* (English edition), 1997; 64:428–431.

Milam, SB, Zardeneta, G, Schmitz, JP. Oxidative stress and degenerative temporomandibular joint disease: a proposed hypothesis. *Journal of Oral and Maxillofacial Surgery*, 1998; 56:214–222.

Mocchegiani, E, Muzzioli, M, Giacconi, R. Zinc and immunoresistance to infection in aging: new biological tools. *Trends Pharmacol Sci*, 2000; 21(6):205–208.

Nelson, HK, Shi, Q, Van Dael, P, et al. Host nutritional selenium status as a driving force for influenza virus mutations. *FASEB Journal*, 2001; 15:1481–1483.

Packer, L. Oxidants, antioxidant nutrients and the athlete. *Journal of Sports Sciences*, 1997; 15:353–363.

Reddy, VN, Giblin, FJ, Lin, L-R, et al. The effect of aqueous humor ascorbate on ultraviolet-B-induced DNA damage in lens epithelium. *Investigative Ophthalmology and Visual Science*, 1998; 39:344–350.

Robinson, K, Arheart, K, Refsum, H, et al. Low circulating folate and vitamin B_6 concentrations. *Circulation*, 1998; 97: 437–443.

Rouault, TA. Iron on the brain. *Nature Genetics*, 2001: 299–300.

Sazawal, S, Black, RE, Jalla, S, et al. Zinc supplementation reduces the incidence of acute lower respiratory infections in infants and preschool children: a double-blind, controlled study. *Pediatrics*, 1998; 102:1–5.

Scott, R, MacPherson, A, Yates, RW, et al. The effect of oral selenium supplementation on human sperm motility. *Br J Urol*, 1998; (1):76–80.

Simon, JA, Grady, D, Snabes, MC, et al. Ascorbic acid supplement use and the prevalence of gallbladder disease. *Journal of Clinical Epidemiology*, 1998; 51: 257–265.

Stephens, NG, Parsons, A, Schofield, PM, et al. Randomised controlled trial of vitamin E in patients with coronary disease: Cambridge Heart Antioxidant Study (CHAOS), *Lancet*, 1996:781–786.

Wang, Hx, Wahlin, A, Basun, H, et al. Vitamin B_{12} and folate in relation to the development of Alzheimer's disease. *Neurology*, 2001; 56:1188–1194.

OTHER BOOKS AND RESOURCES

Balch, JF and Balch, P. *Prescription for Nutritional Healing*, third edition. New York, New York: Avery Penguin Putnam, 2000.

Griffith, H. Winter. *Minerals, Supplements & Vitamins*. Tucson Arizona: Fisher Books, 2000.

Hudson, Tori. *Women's Encyclopedia of Natural Medicine*. Los Angeles, California: Keats Publishing, 1999.

Murray, Michael, and Pizzorno, Joseph. *Encyclopedia of Natural Medicine*, revised second edition. Rocklin, CA: Prima Publishing, 1998.

Redmon, George L. *Minerals What Your Body Really Needs and Why*. Garden City Park, New York: Avery Publishing, 1999.

GreatLife Magazine
Consumer magazine with articles on vitamins, minerals, herbs, and foods.
Available for free at many health and natural food stores.

Let's Live Magazine
Consumer magazine with emphasis on the health benefits of vitamins, minerals, and herbs.
Customer service:
1-800-676-4333
P.O. Box 74908
Los Angeles, CA 90004
Subscriptions: 12 issues per year, $19.95 in the U.S.; $31.95 outside the U.S.

Physical Magazine

Magazine oriented to body builders and other serious athletes.

Customer service:

1-800-676-4333

P.O. Box 74908

Los Angeles, CA 90004

Subscriptions: 12 issues per year, $19.95 in the U.S.; $31.95 outside the U.S.

The Nutrition Reporter™ newsletter

Monthly newsletter that summarizes recent medical research on vitamins, minerals, and herbs.

Customer service:

P.O. Box 30246

Tucson, AZ 85751-0246

e-mail: jack@thenutritionreporter.com

www.nutritionreporter.com

Subscriptions: $26 per year (12 issues) in the U.S.; $32 U.S. or $48 CNC for Canada; $38 for other countries

MEDLINE

http://www.ncbi.nlm.nih.gov/entrez/query

For specific medical journal abstracts.

National Center for Complementary and Alternative Medicine, National Institutes of Health (NIH)

http://nccam.nih.gov/nccam/

Search a database of 180,000 bibliographic citations regarding complementary and alternative therapies extracted from MEDLINE.

Office of Dietary Supplements, National Institutes of Health

http://dietary-supplements.info.nih.gov/

Scientific resources (including recent research findings regarding supplements), general information about supplements, and programs and activities of the Office of Dietary Supplements.

INDEX